HISTOLOGY PRACTICAL HANDBOOK

Chief Editors 吴春云 Ling Eng Ang(林荣安)

Associate Editors 郭泽云 马丽梅 袁 云

Editorial Board Members(Arranged in order of strokes of surname)

U0228551

科学出版社

北 京

内　容　简　介

"HISTOLOGY PRACTICAL HANDBOOK" is a joint effort by several eminent professors from the National University of Singapore and a few leading universities in China. The book contains 196 carefully selected photomicrographs illustrating the four primary basic tissues in histology and the major systems and organs in the body. Each photomicrograph is accompanied by clear and concise descriptive legends highlighting the salient histological features of various tissues and regions. The contents accurately reflect the relevant learning topics and are set at a high level of international standard. Where relevant, they are integrated with human anatomy, pathology, physiology and clinical medicine for the benefit of medical students for their life-long learning, critical thinking and revision of the subject. The book also serves to bridge and strengthen the correlation between different disciplines that is vital to medical professional training.

图书在版编目 (CIP) 数据

HISTOLOGY PRACTICAL HANDBOOK:英文 / 吴春云,(新加坡)林荣安主编 . —北京:科学出版社,2014.1

ISBN 978-7-03-039259-6

Ⅰ. H…　Ⅱ. ①吴… ②林…　Ⅲ. 人体组织学-人体胚胎学-实验-手册-英文　Ⅳ. R329.1-33

中国版本图书馆 CIP 数据核字(2013)第 290688 号

责任编辑:杨鹏远　胡治国 / 责任校对:赵桂芬
责任印制:李　彤 / 封面设计:范璧合

科 学 出 版 社 出版
北京东黄城根北街 16 号
邮政编码:100717
http://www.sciencep.com

北京建宏印刷有限公司 印刷
科学出版社发行　各地新华书店经销

*

2014 年 1 月第 一 版　　开本:787×1092　1/16
2023 年 2 月第五次印刷　　印张:6 1/4
字数:146 000
定价:55.00 元
(如有印装质量问题,我社负责调换)

Preface

As we strive to increase the standards of higher education in our country to match that of international standards, the quality of higher education offered to international students has become an important issue in recent years. Histology, also known as microscopic anatomy, is such that plain observation with the human eye cannot be compared with the intricate details as observed under the microscope. In the latter, practical lessons often serve as an auxiliary teaching method that is deemed to have a direct impact on the study outcomes. This practical guide is therefore aimed to help students to be proficient in this regard. The book is a joint contribution of several eminent histologists from Kunming Medical University, National University of Singapore, Peking University Health Science Center, Sun Yat-Sen University, Capital Medical University, and Huazhong University of Science and Technology. The unique mode of teaching of the discipline is fully reflected in the guide, yet its standard is maintained at a high level with the participation of the leading national and international institutes.

This guide was designed with the following characteristics in mind. Firstly, didactic histology lectures and practical classes are conducted to meet the requirement for professional training of international students. This is possible only through the availability of high quality teaching materials complete with detailed atlas, illustrations and histological explanations. Secondly, the book is co-edited by an eminent professor from the National University of Singapore who has many years of teaching experience in human anatomy and its sub-disciplines. He, together with the local experienced professors, has ensured that the guide is written in acceptable English with strong readability and fluency. Finally, to provide a better understanding between gross anatomy, pathology and clinical presentations, some questions are provided at the end of each chapter to highlight various key aspects of the lesson so as to encourage students to think critically. This will not only assist students to acquire expertise in the subject, but also help them to integrate the topics across various disciplines for clinical applications.

This experimental guide comprises a refined selection of 196 images presented in an order that is consistent with basic theoretical histology teaching. Briefly, it includes light microscopic pictures of the four basic tissues and vital organs of the major organ systems. These images are of high resolution and are described clearly with the use of accompanying labels and text description.

Due to time constraints in coming up with this book, I appeal to your kind understanding for any inadvertent errors or omissions. I therefore urge all readers to provide feedback so that the book may be improved on and perfected for future editions.

Last, but the least, we would like to express our sincere gratitude to the Centre of Experimental Morphology, Kunming Medical University for expert assistance with the photomicrography and immense support.

Wu Chunyun   Ling Eng Ang
October 2013

Contents

Chapter 1　Introduction to Histology Practical Classes and Use of a Light Microscope

Histology is the study of normal microscopic structure of the human or animal body through the light and electron microscopy. In this connection, the practical class is deemed to be the best mode of study to complement as well as enhance the learning of the subject and to better understand and appreciate the functions of the human body at the cellular and tissue levels. Through the microscope, students can on their own better observe and study the morphology of cells, tissues and organs in the laboratory. Indeed, the hands-on practical class is the most efficient way for training of students in their ability for life-long and independent learning, analytical and creative thinking. It is therefore essential for all students to be fully equipped and be competent with the usage of this investigative tool or mode of study.

【Objectives】

　　1. To use the light microscope correctly.

　　2. To describe the structure of cells accurately.

　　3. To know step-by-step the procedure for preparing the paraffin embedded tissue sections and haematoxylin and eosin (H&E) staining routinely used for the practical class.

【Component parts of a light microscope and its usage】

The optical microscope is widely used in different disciplines of science. It plays a vital role for exploration and investigation of tissue organization both in teaching and research. As the microscope is an expensive instrument that demands careful and precise manipulation, any improper usage or poor maintenance may cause damage to the instrument resulting in undesirable outcomes. All students are therefore expected to familiarize yourselves first with the different parts of the microscope and their properties before you intend to examine the microscopic slides independently.

　　1. The basic design of an optical microscope

A standard optical microscope normally consists of two major parts: mechanical component and optical component. The mechanical component includes the stand and arm, ocular tube, nosepiece, specimen stage, specimen holder, focusing device (coarse focus knob and fine focus knob) etc. The optical component includes the eyepiece, the objective lens, condenser, illuminator etc (Figure 1-1).

　　2. How to use a microscope

　　(1) Setting up the microscope: The microscope is an optical instrument with great precision and therefore it should be carefully protected and properly maintained. The placement of the microscope is of utmost important as it should be suitable and comfortable for your own personal observation of slides. For safety reason, it must be kept from the edge of the table at

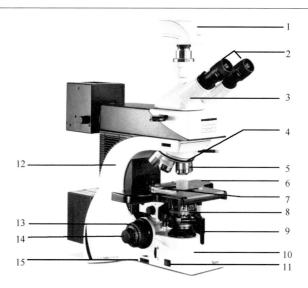

Figure 1-1 Principal parts of an optical microscope

1. Digital camera; 2. Eyepiece; 3. Binocular tube; 4. Nosepiece; 5. Objective lens; 6. Specimen stage; 7. Specimen holder; 8. Condenser; 9. Illuminator; 10. Stand; 11. Power; 12. Arm; 13. Coarse focusing knob; 14. Fine focusing knob; 15. Light control

a distance no less than 6 cm.

(2) Viewing: When viewing a slide with the objective lens, you should always begin with the low-power lens before switching it over to a higher-power lens to avoid damage to the slide or lenses.

A. Use of a low-power objective lens

Turn on the power. Adjust the light path by turning the objective lens to make sure that this maneuver passes through the multiple low-power objective lenses in an ascending order from the lowest power lens. Meanwhile, you should hear a "ka" sound when the objective lens is switched from one to another. Open the diaphragm, raise the condenser and with your two eyes open, adjust the distance between the two oculars. Next, use the illuminative control to allow the optimal lighting. Place a slide on the specimen stage and stabilize it using the specimen holder. Ensure that the tissue section is on the upper side of the slide. Move the specimen into the center of the light path with the thruster and focus on it. Turn the coarse focusing knob to move the stage up to the highest level; then turn the knob slowly to lower the stage. When the image is in the view, turn the fine focusing knob to ensure that it is better focused.

B. Use of a high-power objective lens

Before using the high-power objective lens, you must first find a sharp image under the low-power objective lens. Once you have a selected sharp image under the low-power lens, move the target to the center of the field and focus it. Turn the high-power objective lens very carefully so as not to damage the specimen. Examine the specimen through the ocular by adjusting the fine focusing knob only.

N. B. You should never use the coarse focusing knob under the high power objective lens.

(3) Replacing the glass slides: When you have completed viewing a slide, and would like to move on to the next, you must first move the stage down under the low-power objective lens. After this, remove the slide from the pinchcock in order to avoid damaging to the slide and the objectives.

(4) At the end of the class session, do remember to remove the slide from the microscope, turn off the power, return your microscope to its appropriate place, and put on the dust cover.

3. Additional notes or tips for use of a class microscope

(1) The microscope and the slides must be carefully and properly kept and maintained; the cover slip on a slide placed on the microscope stage should always be face up; changing of slides must be carried out under the low-power objective lens. When using the high-power objective lens, do ensure a safe distance between the objective lens and the slide.

(2) Under no circumstances the lenses are removed from the light microscope. Any loosen or damaged parts should be reported to the teacher-in-charge immediately.

(3) Keep the microscope clean, and any dirt found on it must be wiped off immediately. If the lenses are dirty, clean them gently with a lens paper. Do not use your hands or a handkerchief, or else they may damage the lenses.

(4) Do remember that you are sharing your slide box with other students. After viewing the slides, do make sure to return them to their proper slots. Be considerate.

(5) Before each laboratory class, check the light microscope and the slides. If you notice any damage to the microscope or missing slides, you should report this to the staff-in-charge.

【Procedure for preparation of paraffin embedded tissue sections and H&E staining】

The first step in examination of tissues and organs under a light microscope in the laboratory class is preparation of histology slides. The most commonly used method for this purpose is preparation of tissue sections derived from formalin-fixed tissues which are paraffin-embedded. Tissue sections are first prepared from this and then stained with haematoxylin and eosin (H&E) to differentiate the different components of cells and tissues.

1. Fixation

The purpose of fixation is to prevent the fresh tissue from undergoing autolysis or digestion by bacteria. Fixation preserves the integrity of tissue structure and molecular composition. Some chemical or mixture of chemicals is used as fixatives. Formalin is widely used as a fixative of choice for the preparation of the histology sections. Tissues are usually immersed in solutions of fixatives immediately after they are removed from the body. Before the fixation, the specimen must be cut into the small pieces so as to allow the fixative to penetrate fully into the tissue. Sometimes, the animals such as rats and from which the tissues are derived are perfused by intravascular perfusion. In this case, the fixative can reach the tissue rapidly through the blood vessels (arteries).

2. Paraffin embedding

The purpose of embedding is for obtaining thin tissue sections so that the light can pass through the tissue for optical and optimal visualization under the microscope. The paraffin embedding is used routinely for light microscopy. Before embedding, tissue should be dehydrated with ascending concentrations of alcohol. After this, tissue will be cleared in xylene and impregnated in melted paraffin in the oven which allows the paraffin to diffuse into the tissue spaces. The tissue together with the impregnated paraffin is then solidified outside the oven at room temperature. The hardened blocks containing the tissue are now ready for sectioning on a microtome. Tissue sections are normally cut with a microtome at a thickness ranging from 1 to 10 μm. The sections are floated on water surface and transferred to glass slides to be stained.

3. Staining

To differentiate and better appreciate the different components of tissues and cells, it is necessary to "color" them. Before the staining, paraffin must be dissolved or cleared with xylene. The combination of haematoxylin and eosin (H&E) is the most commonly used staining method. Tissue components that pick up the basic dye are described to be basophilic, while those with an affinity for acid dyes are regarded to be acidophilic.

N. B. Do note that some artifacts such as shrinkage, wrinkles, and precipitates of stain may be present in the slides. These artifacts are linked to the methodology, equipment or reagents used during the preparation process. Students must be aware of the existence of artifacts and appreciate that not every slide in their slide-box collection is always perfect.

【Observation of tissue sections】

1. Neurons, Dorsal root ganglion, H & E

Low power: Many nerve cells (neurons), nerve fibers and glial cells can be seen in the section (Figure 1-2).

High power: The dorsal root ganglion cells or sensory neurons are classified as pseudo-unipolar neurons. The cell body or soma of the neurons is generally round or elliptical. The outline of the neurons is well delineated but the cell membrane (plasma membrane) is not well defined under the microscope. Some bluish granules named Nissl bodies are randomly distributed in the cytoplasm. The nucleus which is often centrally located and bearing

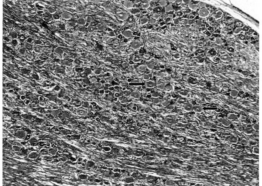

Figure 1-2　Neurons in the dorsal root ganglion, H & E

Black arrows: Neurons

a conspicuous nucleolus is lightly stained. The satellite cells, a form of glial cells, surround the neuronal cell body or soma (Figure 1-3). They provide nutrient support to the neurons.

2. Neurons, Dorsal root ganglion, Silver stain

A section through the dorsal root ganglion stained with silver nitrate. This method facilitates the staining of the Golgi complex of the neurons. The Golgi complex which is stained brown is located in the cytoplasm near the nucleus. Note the nucleus is lightly stained (Figure 1-4). Questions: Why do you think the nucleus of a neuron contains euchromatin predominantly? Name two functions of the Golgi complex.

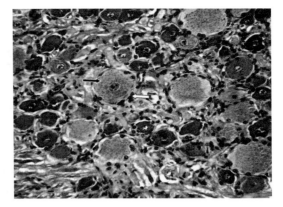

Figure 1-3　Neurons in the dorsal root ganglion, H & E

Black arrow: Neuron; White arrow: Glia cells (satellite cells)

【Demonstration slide】

Glycogen, Liver, PAS (Periodic Acid Schiff) stain

PAS is a histochemical staining that stains glycogen or glycoprotein selectively in cells. Large amounts of particles representing glycogen masses are present in the hepatic cells (Figure 1-5). The nucleus which is palely stained is devoid of glycogen.

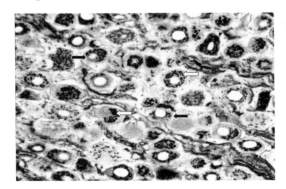

Figure 1-4　Golgi complex in neurons, Silver stain

Black arrows: Neurons; White arrows: Golgi complex

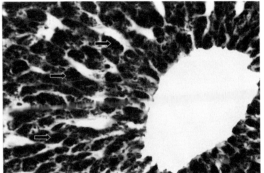

Figure 1-5　Glycogen in hepatic cells, PAS stain

Black arrows: Hepatocytes

【Questions】

1. What is basophilia? What is acidophilia?

2. Which histological staining is routinely used for study of cells and tissues?

3. Using the neuron as an example, describe the light microscopic structure of a cell.

(郭泽云)

Chapter 2　Epithelial Tissue

Epithelial tissue is avascular; it covers the body surface, lines the body cavities and constitutes glands. The tissue is composed of closely aggregated cells with very little extracellular matrix. The epithelial cells show a polarity having free, lateral and basal surfaces. There are three types of epithelial tissue including the covering epithelium, glandular epithelium and special epithelium. The principal functions of epithelium are protection, absorption, secretion, and sensory reception.

【Objectives】

　　1. To identify and describe:

　　A. simple squamous epithelium.

　　B. simple cuboidal epithelium.

　　C. simple columnar epithelium.

　　D. pseudostratified ciliated columnar epithelium.

　　E. stratified squamous (keratinized and nonkeratinized).

　　2. To understand the main features and functions of the transitional epithelium.

【Observation of tissue sections】

　　1. Simple squamous epithelium, Kidney, H & E

Naked eye: The tissue section appears pyramidal in outline. The area close to the base of the pyramid is the cortex of the kidney; nearer to the apex of the pyramid is the medulla.

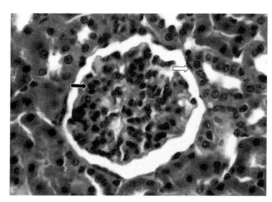

**Figure 2-1　Simple squamous epithelium,
Kidney, H & E**

Black arrow: Renal corpuscle; White arrow: Simple
squamous epithelium

Low power: Many renal corpuscles are distributed in the cortex. Identify the renal corpuscles and focus on one of them.

High power: A renal corpuscle comprises the glomerulus and the renal capsule (Bowman's capsule). Note that the parietal layer of the renal capsule is lined by simple squamous epithelium. In the latter, the squamous cells are polygonal in shape on a surface view but appear flattened and very thin on a side view. They appear as a cellular sheet under the light microscope (Figure 2-1).

　　2. Simple cuboidal epithelium, Kidney, H & E

Low power: Examine the medulla of the kidney. Many collecting tubules may be seen.

Focus on these tubules.

High power: The collecting tubule is lined by simple cuboidal epithelium (Figure 2-2) composed of cells with a square profile; often, the height of the cells is slightly greater than the width. These cells have a round and centrally located nucleus.

3. Simple columnar epithelium, Gall bladder, H & E

Low power: Simple columnar epithelium lines the lumen of the gall bladder.

High power: The cells are tall and the nuclei are located in the basal area of the cells. Note the distinct striated border which is formed by large, uniform microvilli present on the free surface of the cells (Figure 2-3).

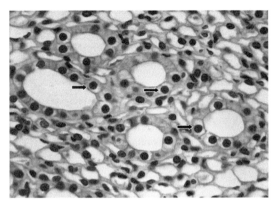

Figure 2-2   Simple cubodial epithelium,
Kidney, H & E

Black arrows: Simple cuboidal epithelium

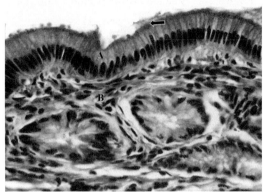

Figure 2-3   Simple columnar epithelium,
Gall bladder, H & E

A: Simple columnar epithelium; B: Connective
tissue; Black arrow: Striated border

4. Pseudostratified ciliated columnar epithelium, Trachea, H & E

Low power: The internal or luminal surface of the trachea is lined by ciliated pseudostratified columnar epithelium also called the respiratory epithelium.

High power: The epithelium is composed of more than one type of epithelial cells which vary in sizes and heights. Not all the constituent cells reach the surface but all are adhered to the basement membrane. In view of this, the nuclei are located at different levels in a sectional profile. These features give the epithelium a false impression of stratification. It is actually a simple epithelium. Identify the columnar cells and the goblet cells. The columnar cell has cilia at its apical surface. The goblet cell stains pale. Some cells on the bottom of the epithelium are the small basal cells (Figure 2-4). Question: What is the specific function of the respective cell types?

5. Nonkeratinized stratified squamous epithelium, Esophagus, H & E

Low power: the esophagus is lined by nonkeratinized stratified squamous epithelium (Figure 2-5).

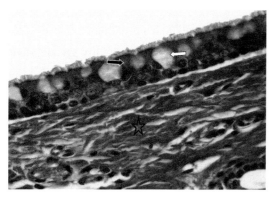

Figure 2-4   Pseudostratified cilia columnar epithelium, Trachea, H & E

Black arrow: Columnar cell; White arrow: Goblet cell; Asterisk: Connective tissue

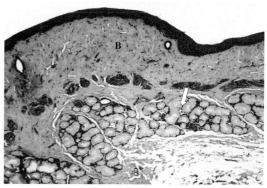

Figure 2-5   Nonkeratinized stratified squamous epithelium, Esophagus, H & E

A: Epithelium; B: Connective tissue; White arrow: Esophageal glands

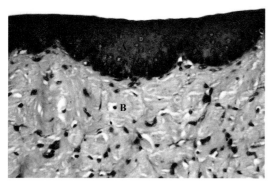

Figure 2-6   Nonkeratinized stratified squamous epithelium, Esophagus, H & E

A: Epithelium; B: Connective tissue

High power: nonkeratinized stratified squamous epithelium is composed of multi-layered cells. Its name derives from the shape of the outer layer of flattened cells. Note that all the squamous cells retain nuclei and lack the keratin. The surface cells are flattened. In the middle layer, the cells are polyhedral. The basal layer consists of a row of cells bearing somewhat oval nuclei indicating that the shape of cells is low columnar (Figure 2-6).

6. Keratinized stratified squamous epithelium, Skin, H & E

Low power: The superficial layer is the epidermis of the skin and the area beneath the epithelium is dermis. Identify the epidermis which consists of the keratinized stratified squamous epithelium (Figure 2-7).

High power: The keratinized stratified squamous epithelium also consists of multilayered cells. The cells closer to the underlying connective tissue are usually cuboidal or columnar. The cells assume an irregular and flattened outline as they move progressively closer to the surface, where they are thin and squamous. The superficial cells are dead cells containing the keratin and lacking nuclei (Figure 2-8).

Differentiate the nonkeratinized stratified squamous epithelium from the keratinized stratified squamous epithelium. What are their major histological differences?

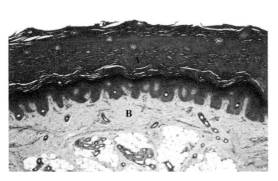

Figure 2-7 Keratinized stratified squamous epithelium, Skin, H & E

A: Epidermis; B: Dermis

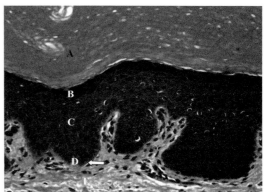

Figure 2-8 Keratinized stratified squamous epithelium, Skin, H & E

A: Keratinized dead cells; B: Flatted cells; C: Polyhedral cells; D: Low columnar cells; E: Connective tissue; White arrow: Basement membrane

【Demonstration slides】

1. Simple squamous epithelium, Mesentery, Silver stain

The epithelium is composed of squamous cells. The cell boundaries are delineated by dark silver staining. The cells are flattened, generally polygonal in shape (Figure 2-9).

2. Transitional epithelium (also called the urothelium as it is confined to the urinary system), Bladder, H & E

Transitional epithelium lines the surface of the bladder. Compare the structure of the transitional epithelium when the urinary bladder is empty (Figure 2-10)

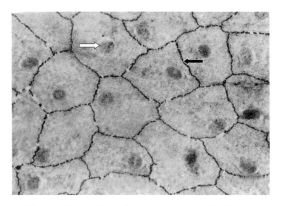

Figure 2-9 Simple squamous epithelium, Silver stain

Black arrow: Boundary of cells; White arrow: Nucleus

and when it is full (Figure 2-11). When the bladder is empty (relaxed state), the epithelium is normally 4 ~ 6 cell-layered thick; the cells in the top layer appear dome-shaped and are referred to as the "facet cells". Sometimes, the "facet cells" show two containing nuclei which are therefore bi-nucleated. When the bladder is full (distended state), the top dome-shaped cells become flattened and the epithelium becomes thinner.

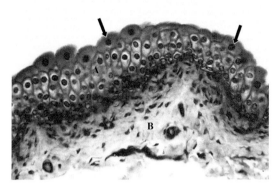

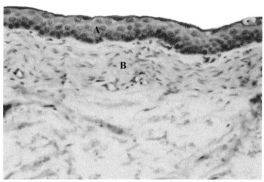

Figure 2-10   Transitional epithelium, Bladder（relaxed state）, H & E

A: Epithelium; B: Connective tissue; Black arrows: Facet cells

Figure 2-11   Transitional epithelium, Bladder（distended state）, H & E

A: Epithelium; B: Connective tissue

【Questions】

1. Name the lining epithelium of the following tissues/structures /organs: esophagus, ileum, vagina, peritoneal cavity, pulmonary alveolus, nasopharynx and arteries.

2. Name the common types of cell junctions between epithelial cells and what are their functions?

3. What are the differences in structure of cilia, microvilli and stereocilia?

（郭泽云）

Chapter 3　Connective Tissue Proper

Connective tissue consists of cells and the extracellular matrix which contains fibers and amorphous ground substance. Unlike the other tissues (epithelium, muscle, and nerve tissue), which are formed mainly by cells, the major constituent of the connective tissue is the extracellular matrix. The connective tissue encompasses connective tissue proper and specialized cartilage, bone and blood. There are four types of connective tissue proper including the loose connective tissue, dense connective tissue, adipose tissue and reticular tissue. Several types of cells are present in the connective tissue. They are fibroblasts, mast cells, macrophages, plasma cells, adipocytes and leucocytes. The function of the connective tissue is to provide form and structural support to the body and organs. It is also a medium for exchange of nutrients, oxygen, and waste products between other tissues. Meanwhile, they have also defense and repairing roles.

【Objectives】

1. To identify and describe:

A. the fibroblasts, macrophages, collagen and elastic fibers.

B. the basic structure of loose connective tissue, dense connective tissue and adipose tissue.

2. To understand and describe briefly the structure and function of mast cell, plasma cell, reticular cell and reticular fiber.

【Observation of tissue sections】

1. Loose connective tissue, Teased preparation of mesentery, Special stain

Low power: Some dark blue / purple squiggly fibers (elastic fibers), larger straight pink fibers (collagen), and cells may be seen in the section. The fibers provide the basic structural framework of the loose connective tissue. A variety of cells are distributed in the ground substance.

High power: The elastic fibers are thin and squiggly while the collagen fibers are thick and straight. Are you able to distinguish the fibroblast from the macrophage? The macrophages are identifiable by the contents of ingested materials (trypan blue dye) in the cytoplasm. It is difficult to identify precisely the cell outline of the fibroblast. Under the light microscope, the cells are normally oval-shaped or rounded and show a lightly stained nucleus (Figure 3-1).

2. Loose connective tissue, Stomach, H & E

Low power: Stomach is composed of four layers: mucosa, submucosa, muscularis externa and adventitia. The submuscosa consists of the loose connective tissue (Figure 3-2).

High power: The loose connective tissue is "loosely organized in texture" as the name implies. The containing interlacing fibers composed of collagen and elastic fibers are difficult

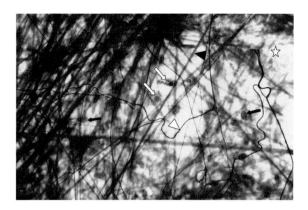

Figure 3-1 Loose connective tissue, Special stain

Black arrows: Fibroblasts; White arrows: Macrophages; Black arrowhead: Collagen fiber; White
arrowhead: Elastic fiber; Asterisk: Ground substance

to distinguish with the H&E staining. The rich ground substance is lightly stained and embedded in it are the variety of connective tissue cells, the majority of them being fibroblasts/fibro-
cytes. In addition, many blood vessels may be seen traversing the loose connective tissue
(Figure 3-3).

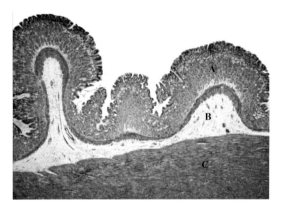

Figure 3-2 Loose connective tissue, H & E

A: Mucosa; B: Submucosa (loose connective
tissue); C: Muscularis externa

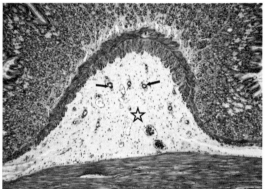

Figure 3-3 Loose connective tissue, H & E

Asterisk: Loose connective tissue; Black arrows:
Blood vessels

3. Dense irregular connective tissue, Skin, H & E

Low power: The dermis lies beneath the keratinized stratified squamous epithelium and it
is made up of the dense irregular connective tissue (Figure 3-4).

High power: Dense irregular connective tissue contains many randomly oriented bundles
of collagen fibers. These collagen fibers are thick and are densely arranged. Between the
densely organized fibers are sparsely distributed cells (mainly fibrocytes/fibroblasts) and the
ground substance (Figure 3-5).

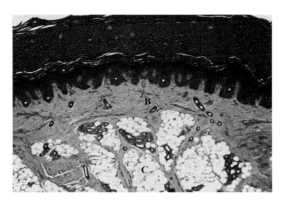

Figure 3-4   Dense irregular connective tissue, Skin, H & E

A: Epidermis; B: Dermis (dense irregular connective tissue); C: Adipose tissue

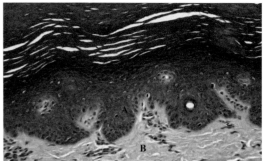

Figure 3-5   Dense irregular connective tissue, Skin, H & E

A: Keratinized stratified squamous epithelium; B: Dense irregular connective tissue

4. Adipose tissue, Skin, H & E

Low power: Many empty looking cells which are stained very lightly are seen beneath the dense connective tissue. These cells are adipocytes. The adipose tissue often exists in locules is composed of closely packed adipocytes (Figure 3-4).

High power: The adipocytes are round cells. The cell contains a large droplet of lipid in the cytoplasm which was dissolved in the process of tissue embedding and staining. This has resulted in an achromatic color ("empty looking") (Figure 3-6). The nucleus of the adipocyte is pressed against the periphery of

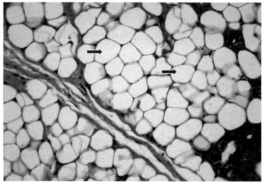

Figure 3-6   Adipose tissue, Skin, H & E

Black arrows: Adipocytes

the cell. Surrounding the adipocytes is the connective tissue.

【Demonstration slides】

1. Plasma cells, H & E

The plasma cells are characterized by a clock-face nucleus and basophilic cytoplasm (Figure 3-7). (N. B. The basophilia is due to the well-developed rough endoplasmic reticulum as required by the cell for protein synthesis-immunoglobulins).

2. Mast cells, Toluidine blue stain

The mast cells have a single oval nucleus and large amounts of granules in its cytoplasm (Figure 3-8). The cytoplasmic granules cannot be stained with H&E, but they appear purple in section stained with toluidine blue. This unique histochemical staining phenomenon is called metachromasia indicating that the granules are rich in acid mucopolysaccharide. Question: What is the main secretion of mast cells? Name the actions of the secretion.

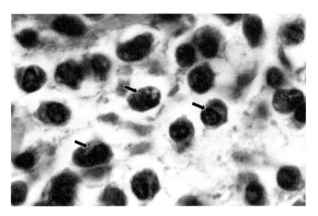

Figure 3-7   Plasma cells, H & E

Black arrows: Plasma cells

3. Reticular fibers, Liver, Silver stain

Reticular fibers are darkly stained and appear extremely branched with the silver staining (Figure 3-9). The fibers form a stromal network supporting the framework of the organ. (N. B. the dark staining of the reticular fibers is due to the rich amounts of carbohydrates associated with them and this is a distinguishing feature from the collagen fibers). The reticular fibers have a staining affinity for silver which is therefore described to be "agyrophilic".

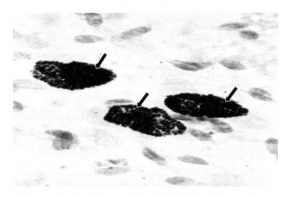

Figure 3-8   Mast cells, Toluidine blue stain

Black arrows: Mast cells

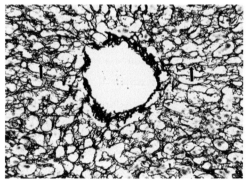

Figure 3-9   Reticular fibers, Liver, Silver stain

Black arrows: Reticular fibers

【Questions】

1. Using the dermis (dermal papilla) as an example, describe the cell types and intercellular matrix (fibers and ground substance) of the loose connective tissue.

2. Describe the structure and functions of the following cell types: mast cells, macrophages, fibroblasts and adipocytes (fat cells).

3. Describe the molecular mechanism of biosynthesis of collagen fibril.

4. Describe the histological features of tendon e. g. biceps tendon.

(郭小兵 赵 敏)

Chapter 4   Cartilage and Bone

Cartilage and bone are specialized form of connective tissue which plays a critical role in providing a structural framework of the body without which the body would collapse. Cartilage is characterized by its main constituent cells, namely, chondrocytes distributed in cell clusters and embedded in an extracellular matrix rich in glycosaminoglycans and proteoglycans which are macromolecules that cross-link with collagen and elastic fibers. There are three types of cartilage: hyaline cartilage, fibrocartilage and elastic cartilage, differ mostly in histologic appearance and properties of extracellular matrix in terms of amounts and nature of fibers. Bone tissue is composed of its constituent cells and between them is the body matrix which as a rigid connective tissue consists of massive collagen embedded in a ground substance. The ground substance is impregnated with inorganic calcium phosphate that is deposited or associated with the collagen between osteocytes. There are three main types of constituent cells in the bone tissue: osteoblasts, osteocytes and osteoclasts.

【Objectives】

1. To identify and describe:

A. hyaline cartilage, chondrocytes, lacuna, isogenic cell group.

B. haversian system (osteon), interstitial lamella, lacuna, canaliculi.

2. To understand and describe:

A. the histological differences between hyaline cartilage, fibrocartilage and elastic cartilage.

B. the differences between endochondral and intramembranous ossification.

【Observation of tissue sections】

1. Hyaline cartilage, Trachea, H & E

Low power: Note the C-shaped hyaline cartilage which partially circles the trachea thus keeping its lumen patent. It constitutes the major part of the outermost tunic (adventitia) of the trachea (Figure 4-1).

High power: The hyaline cartilage is composed of the chondrocytes and extracellular matrix. The extracellular matrix may be stained bluish or light purple, which includes the territorial matrix and interterritorial matrix (territorial matrix is stained darker than interterritorial matrix) (Figure 4-2). The chondrocytes are located in the lacuna. The cells near the perichondrium (the covering of cartilage) are flattened, while those in the deeper zones are more rounded. Isogenic cell groups are common in mature hyaline cartilage. The collagen fibrils embedded in the ground substance are not identifiable as the refractive index is similar to that of the ground substance. The hyaline cartilage is an avascular tissue which is nourished by diffusion of nutrients from the perichondrium composed of connective tissue with blood vessels.

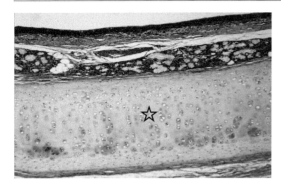

Figure 4-1   Hyaline cartilage, Trachea,
H & E

Asterisk: Hyaline cartilage

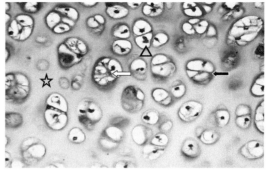

Figure 4-2   Hyaline cartilage, Trachea,H & E

Asterisk: Interterritorial matrix; Black arrow: Territorial matrix; White arrow: Isogenic cell group; Arrowhead: Chondrocyte

2. Compact bone, Femoral bone, Silver stain

Low power: This is a transverse section of the femur showing the compact bone. The outer circumferential lamellae and inner circumferential lamellae are not included in this section.
Numerous Haversian systems (osteons) are shown in the compact bone. There are also
present some interstitial lamellae between the osteons (Figure 4-3).

High power: An osteon is made up of a central Harversian canal surrounded by 4 ~ 20
concentric bony lamellae. Note each osteocyte is housed in a lacuna showing a variable number of radiating canaliculi (Figure 4-4). Note also that the canaliculi from adjacent lacunae
have direct communication. By this configuration, osteocytes in the lacunae are making end-
to-end contacts via gap junctions at the tip of their processes lying in the canaliculi.

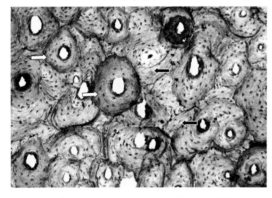

Figure 4-3   Compact bone, Femoral bone,
Silver stain

White arrows: Osteons; Black arrows: Interstitial
lamellae

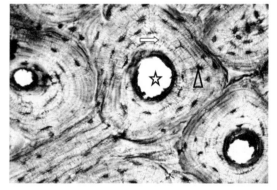

Figure 4-4   Osteons, Compact bone,
Silver stain

White arrow: Canaliculi; Arrowhead:Bone lacuna;
Asterisk:Harversian canal

【Demonstration slides】

1. Elastic cartilage in epiglottis, Special stain

Elastic cartilage contains darkly stained elastic fibers forming a dense, closely packed meshwork (Figure 4-5). The elastic fibers provide elasticity to this tissue. The other characteristic features resemble that of the hyaline cartilage.

2. Fibrocartilage, H & E

The fibrocartilage contains abundant collagen fibers (Figure 4-6); hence, the matrix is eosinophilic. There are fewer chondrocytes which are arranged in parallel cell columns or rows compared with the hyaline cartilage.

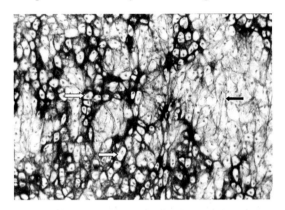

Figure 4-5   Elastic cartilage, Special stain

Black arrow: Elastic fibers; White arrows: Chondrocytes

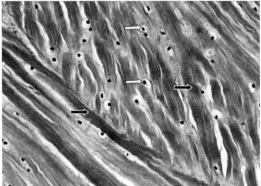

Figure 4-6   Fibrocartilage, H & E

Black arrows: Collagen fibers; White arrows: Chondrocytes

3. Osteoblasts and osteoclasts, H & E

The osteoblasts are cuboidal or columnar in shape with a basophilic cytoplasm. The cells are aligned in rows along the surface of the bone matrix (Figure 4-7). Osteoblasts are responsible for the synthesis of osteoid (prebone) and induce matrix mineralization during the bone development and remodeling.

An osteoclast, lying in a bony depression "Howship's lacuna", is a large cell with several nuclei and a ruffled cell border opposing the bone matrix (Figure 4-8). It is responsible for bone resorption and remodeling via secretion of collagenase and hydrolytic enzymes. The site of osteoclastic activity is evidenced by a bony depression called the Howship's lacuna.

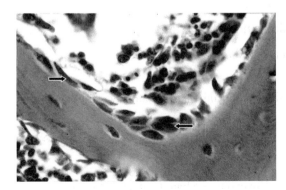

Figure 4-7   Osteoblasts, H & E

Black arrows: Osteoblasts

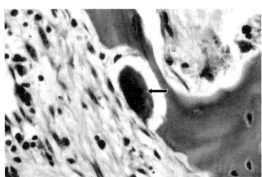

Figure 4-8   Osteoclast, H & E

Black arrow: Osteoclast

4. Cartilaginous (Endochondral) ossification, Phalanx of a human fetus, H & E

Lower power: The primary ossification center is located in the center of each phalanx which contains a marrow cavity, collections of immature blood cells, and many bony trabeculae. From the epiphysial to the diaphysial side, the following cell zones may be identified (Figure 4-9, Figure 4-10).

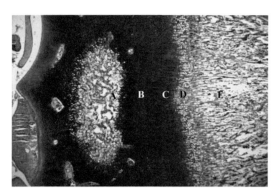

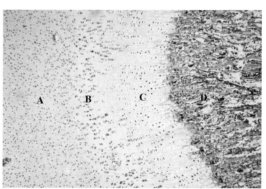

Figure 4-9 Cartilaginous (Endochondral) ossification, H & E

A: Secondary ossification center; B: Resting zone; C: Proliferative zone; D: Calcified cartilage zone; E: Ossification zone

Figure 4-10 Cartilaginous (Endochondral) ossification, H & E

A: Resting zone; B: Proliferative zone; C: Calcified cartilage zone; D: Ossificaton zone

(1) Resting zone: It consists of hyaline cartilage with small chondrocytes and pale matrix.

(2) Proliferative zone: Chondrocytes undergo rapid mitosis. Cells are stacked into columns and are parallel to the long axis of future bone.

(3) Calcified cartilage zone: Chondrocytes are hypertrophied and gradually degenerate and die. Cartilage matrix becomes calcified and stained dark-blue.

(4) Ossification zone: Remnants of calcified cartilage matrix are covered by red staining bone tissue forming the mixed trabeculae or spicules.

【Questions and clinical points for discussion and integration】

1. Compare the histological differences between the three types of cartilage. Give an example of each of the cartilage types.

2. Describe the microscopic structure of the epiphysial plate. Name two hormones that may act on its growth.

3. Describe the histological features of intramembranous ossification using the skull bone e. g. frontal or parietal bone as an example.

4. Describe the histological structure of a Haversian system (osteon) in the compact bone of a mature long bone.

5. Describe the following cell types in terms of their structure and functions: osteocyte, osteoblast and osteoclast. What is the origin of osteoclast? How do you distinguish it from a megakaryocyte present in the red bone marrow?

6. Describe the microscopic structure of hyaline cartilage. What is the mode of its growth?

7. Give an account of the histological differences between endochondral and intramembranous ossification.

（杨　力）

Chapter 5　Blood

Blood can be regarded as the fluid tissue which circulates through the cardiovascular system. It is a specialized type of connective tissue, composed of cells, cell fragments, and plasma which is an extracellular fluid element. The formed cells and cell fragments of blood are erythrocytes (red blood cells, RBCs), leukocytes (white blood cells, WBCs), and platelets. The functions of erythrocytes are entirely within the circulatory system by transporting O_2 from lungs to tissues and returning CO_2 from tissues to lungs for elimination. Leukocytes perform their functions outside the circulatory system and use the bloodstream as a mode of transportation to reach their destinations. There are two major categories of leukocytes: agranulocytes and granulocytes. The first group comprises lymphocytes and monocytes, and the second group is composed of neutrophils, eosinophils, and basophils.

【Objectives】

1. To identify and describe:

A. the light microscopic structure of erythrocytes and platelets.

B. the light microscopic structure of five types of leukocytes. You should be able to identify the neutrophils, eosinophils, basophils, lymphocytes, and monocytes.

2. To understand and describe the light microscopic structure of reticulocytes.

【Observation of tissue section】

Blood smear, Wright's stain

The erythrocytes far outnumber the platelets and they, in turn, are much more numerous than the white blood cells. Based on morphological criteria and under the higher magnification (Figure 5-1), differentiate the following blood cells and, where possible, examine the cells in detail under the oil immersion lens.

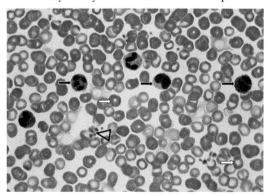

Figure 5-1　Blood smear, Wright's stain

Black arrows: Leukocytes; White arrows: Erythrocytes;
Arrowhead: Platelets

1. **Erythrocytes** measuring 7 to 10 μm in diameter; anucleate (lacking a nucleus); rounded and biconcave disc (Figure 5-1).

Erythrocyte displays a central clear, pale region that represents the thinnest area of the biconcave disc, while the peripheral zone of erythrocyte is stained deep orange-red. The size of the central zone and the overall staining intensity of the erythrocyte are proportional to the content of haemoglobin.

　　2. **Platelets**　measuring 2 to 4 μm in diameter; anucleate; oval-to-round fragments (Figure 5-1). Platelets are cytoplasmic fragments derived from megakaryocytes of the bone marrow. As such, they possess no nuclei, and are frequently clumped together. They present with a dark blue, central granular region, the granulomere, and a light blue, peripheral, clear region, the hyalomere.

　　3. **Leukocytes**　nucleate, rounded (Figure 5-1).

　　The number of leukocytes is much smaller than that of erythrocytes. The leukocytes are classified into two groups based on the contents of the specific granules.

　　(1) Granulocytes: They are recognizable by their distinctive specific granules, whose coloration provides the classification for three different types of leukocytes; another distinguishing feature is the presence of a multi-lobed nucleus.

　　• Neutrophils: measuring 9 to 12 μm in diameter (Figure 5-2).

　　Neutrophils are the most numerous in all leukocytes. They constitute about 50% to 70% of total leukocyte count, and are therefore the easiest cells to identify amongst the 5 types of leukocytes. These cells display a light pink cytoplasm laden with many azurophilic and smaller specific granules. Large azurophilic granules (affinity for Azure A stain which is a metachromatic stain) are stained reddish purple, while many small, membrane-bound specific granules are neither acidophilic nor basophilic but are stained faintly with neutral dyes. The nucleus is dark blue and multilobed, mostly two to three-lobed; the lobes are interconnected by thin strands. Neutrophils are avid phagocytes—scavenger cells which have the capability to engulf bacteria, cell debris, and foreign matter. The number of neutrophils is markedly increased in acute bacterial infections.

　　• Eosinophils: measuring 12 to 15 μm in diameter (Figure 5-3).

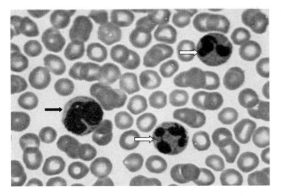 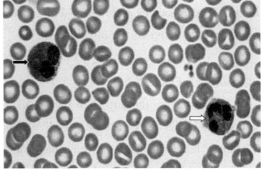

Figure 5-2　Blood smear, Wright's stain
Black arrow: Monocyte; White arrows: Neutrophils

Figure 5-3　Blood smear, Wright's stain
Black arrow: Eosinophil; White arrow: Neutrophil

　　Eosinophils constitute 1% to 4% of total leukocyte count. They are slightly larger than the neutrophils. These cells show a granular cytoplasm full of brightly stained large, red-orange specific granules and a bilobed (two lobes) nucleus. The functions of eosinophils are to eliminate antigen-antibody complexes, and to destroy parasitic worms. Elevated cell numbers occur in parasitic infections and allergic responses such as hay fever and asthma.

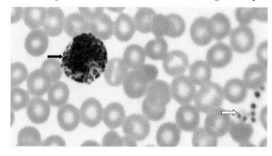

Figure 5-4　Blood smear, Wright's stain
Black arrow: Basophil; White arrow: Platelets

• Basophils: measuring 10 to 14 μm in diameter (Figure 5-4).

Basophils are the least numerous amongst the leukocytes. They account for less than 1% of total leukocytes count and are therefore more difficult to find in a routine blood smear. Frequently, their cytoplasm is so filled with large, distinctive basophilic specific granules that they appear to mask the nucleus which is often irregular in shape or bilobed. Basophils function as initiators of the inflammatory process and they play an important role in initiation of allergic reactions. The number of basophils increases in many clinical conditions such as hay fever, urticaria, chronic sinusitis, and some leukemia.

（2）Agranulocytes

• Lymphocytes: small-sized cells, measuring 6 to 10 μm in diameter (Figure 5-5); medium-to large-sized cells, measuring 11 to 16 μm in diameter.

Lymphocytes constitute 20% ~ 30% of the total circulating leukocyte count. They are round cells in blood smear, and are usually same as or somewhat larger size than erythrocytes. Most circulating lymphocytes in normal blood are small. These spherical cells have a thin rim of blue-gray cytoplasm. The densely stained and round nucleus, with a great deal of heterochromatin, is often eccentrically placed. Question: What is the difference between heterochromatin and euchromatin? Lymphocytes can be subdivided into three functional categories, namely T lymphocytes which constitute 60% ~ 80% of lymphocytes in normal peripheral blood; B lymphocytes and natural killer (NK) cells. Morphologically they are indistinguishable from each other in the blood smear.

• Monocytes: measuring 12 to 20 μm in diameter (Figure 5-5).

Monocytes are the largest in the circulating blood cells and constitute 3% ~ 8% of the total leukocyte count. They have a lightly stained, eccentric nucleus that often appears as horseshoe or kidney-shaped. The cytoplasm is bluish gray and has some azurophilic granules and occasional vacuole-like spaces. Monocytes can cross walls of venules and capillaries through a process

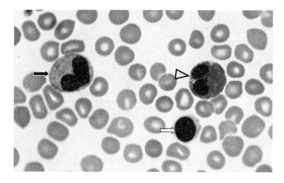

Figure 5-5　Blood smear, Wright's stain
Black arrow: Monocyte; White arrow: Lymphocyte;
Arrowhead: Eosinophil

called "diapedesis" and become macrophages including histiocytes (connective tissue), alveolar and peritoneal macrophages, Kupffer cells in the liver and microglia in the brain constituting the so-called Mononuclear Phagocyte System. Large numbers of monocytes infiltrate areas of inflammation, where they are actively engaged in phagocytosis, scavenging of cell debris and releasing poinflammatory cytokines such as tumor necrosis factor-alpha (TNF-α) and interleukin-1 beta (IL-1β).

【Demonstration slide】

Reticulocyte, Blood smear, Brilliant cresyl blue stain

Reticulocytes normally account for less than 1% of the total erythrocyte population. They resemble normal, circulating erythrocytes but lacking a nucleus. When stained with brilliant cresyl blue in a blood smear, however, a bluish reticulum (Figure 5-6)— composed mostly of rough endoplasmic reticulum—is evident. Reticulocytes are larger than mature erythrocytes, measuring approximately 9 μm in diameter.

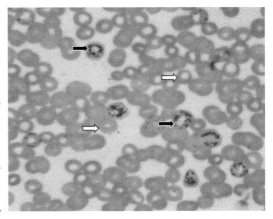

Figure 5-6　Reticulocyte, Brilliant cresyl blue stain

Black arrows: Reticulocytes; White arrows: Erythrocytes

【Questions】

1. Describe the features and functions of the erythrocytes.

2. Describe the identifying features of various leukocytes as seen in a blood smear preparation.

（唐军民　马丽梅）

Chapter 6   Muscle Tissue

There are three types of muscle tissue whose classification is based on histological and functional differences. Functionally, muscle is either under the control at will (voluntary muscle) or is not (involuntary muscle). Structurally, it either shows regular transverse bands along the length of the fibers (striated muscle) or does not (smooth, or unstriated muscle). On this basis, the three types of muscle are as follows.

1. Striated voluntary or skeletal muscle: It is attached to bones or fascia and constitutes the "flesh" or "muscle" of the limbs and body wall. The contraction is powerful and rapid.

2. Striated involuntary or cardiac muscle: It forms the wall of the heart; it is also distributed in the walls of major blood vessels.

3. Smooth involuntary muscle: It is present in the walls of the hollow viscus and most blood vessels. Contraction is slow and sluggish.

This practical class is aimed to study the light microscopic structure of the three types of muscle, but more importantly, with the knowledge gained you should be able to relate this to their primary physiological function-muscle contraction.

【Objectives】

To identify and describe the light microscopic structure of the skeletal, cardiac and smooth muscle fibers and highlight their major differences.

【Observation of tissue sections】

1. Skeletal muscle, H & E

This slide contains two tissue sections of skeletal muscle: a longitudinal and a transverse section. In a longitudinal section (Figure 6-1), the muscle fibers are long and cylindrical so that both ends of the fibers are not included in the section. Between the muscle fibers is a small amount of delicate connective tissue, the endomysium. At a higher magnification, the skeletal muscle fibers are multinucleated cells whose nuclei are located at the periphery of the fiber. There are two types of striations in the skeletal muscle cells, longitudinal and transverse. The longitudinal striations represent the myofibrils, which are not clearly defined. The transverse striations are more conspicuous, as manif-

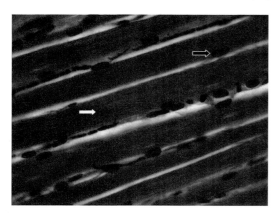

Figure 6-1   Skeletal muscle (longitudinal), H & E

White arrow: Skeletal muscle fiber; Black arrow: Nucleus

ested by the alternate dark (A) and light (I) transverse bands due to the regular and staggering arrangement of the myofibrils, or contractile protein filaments. Locate the A and I bands of the muscle fibers. Question: What is the basic contractile unit of skeletal muscle and what it its structure?

Skeletal muscle fibers as seen in a transverse section (Figure 6-2). Note the constituent muscle fibers which appear as eosinophilic polygonal profiles. The cut ends of the myofibrils give the cut surface a stippled appearance. The peripheral location

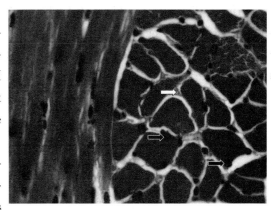

Figure 6-2   Skeletal muscle (transverse), H & E

Black arrows: Nuclei; White arrow: Endomysium

of the nuclei is evident in a cross sectional profile of the muscle fibers. The endomysium is closely associated with the individual muscle fibers or lies between them.

2. Cardiac muscle, H & E
3. Cardiac muscle, Special stain

The muscle bundles in the heart are organized in different orientations. Survey the section at low magnification and by doing so you should be able to identify the muscle fibers either in longitudinal (Figure 6-3, Figure 6-4) or in transverse sections (Figure 6-5, Figure 6-6). Cardiac muscle fibers show striations, but they are not as obvious as in the skeletal muscle fibers in longitudinal sections. These fibers (cells) are branched, varying in diameter, and have a centrally located nucleus. An intercalated disc (black arrow, Figure 6-3, Figure 6-4), which represents the site of intercellular junction between two cardiac muscle fibers, appears as a distinct dark line in the light micrographs. What are the distinctive features of an intercalated disc in the electron micrograph?

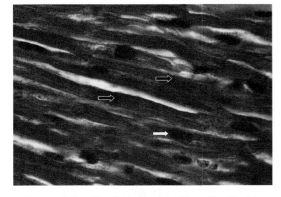

Figure 6-3   Cardiac muscle (longitudinal), H & E

Black arrows: Intercalated discs; White arrow: Nucleus

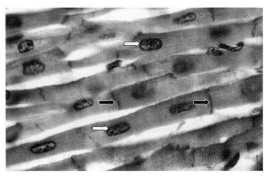

Figure 6-4   Cardiac muscle (longitudinal), Special stain

Black arrows: Intercalated discs; White arrows: Nuclei

The cardiac muscle (Figure 6-5, Figure 6-6) in a transverse sectional view demonstrates the polygonal shape of its muscle fibers. The nucleus of each muscle cell (fiber) is located in the center, but not all cells display a nucleus (Explain this). In a transverse section, myofibrils may be recognizable as numerous small dots of varying diameters within the sarcoplasm. Are intercalated discs identifiable in a transverse section of the muscle fiber?

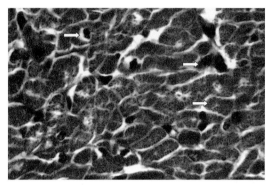 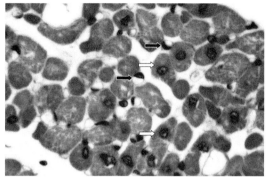

**Figure 6-5　Cardiac muscle (transverse),
H & E**

White arrows: Cardiac muscle fibers

**Figure 6-6　Cardiac muscle (transverse),
Special stain**

Black arrows: Capillaries; White arrows: Cardiac
muscle fibers

4. Smooth muscle, H & E

The muscle fibers in the intestine run in various directions; therefore, some of the fibers are cut longitudinally (B, Figure 6-7), while others are sectioned transversely (A, Figure 6-7), and still others are cut obliquely. In a longitudinal section, the smooth muscle is made up of long fusiform smooth muscle fibers (white arrow, Figure 6-8) with a centrally located, elongated nucleus (black arrow, Figure 6-8). Since the muscle fibers are arranged in staggered arrays, they are closely packed and as such only a limited amount of intervening connective tissue exists.

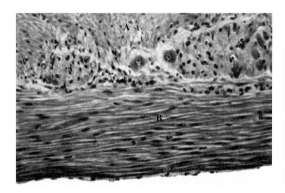 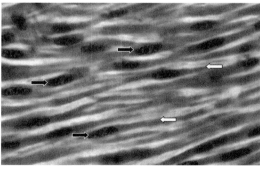

Figure 6-7　Smooth muscle, H & E

A: Transverse section; B: Longitudinal section

**Figure 6-8　Smooth muscle (longitudinal),
H & E**

White arrows: Smooth muscle fibers; Black arrows:
Nuclei

Note that the profiles of the smooth muscle cells in a transverse section vary in size (Figure 6-9). The round nucleus is surrounded by a thin rim of cytoplasm. If the nucleus were to be sectioned at its tapered end, only a small dot of it would be present in the center of a large muscle fiber. Additionally, the cell may be sectioned in a region away from its nucleus, where only the sarcoplasm of the large muscle cell would be evident.

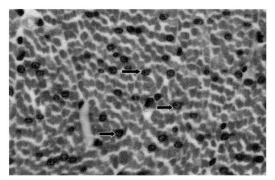

**Figure 6-9   Smooth muscle (transverse),
H & E**

Black arrows: Round nuclei

【Questions and topics for discussion and integration】

1. Compare and contrast the histological features between the skeletal muscle and cardiac muscle.

2. Describe the structure of a sarcomere in the skeletal muscle fiber as seen under the electron microscope.

3. What are the major histological differences between the cardiac muscle and smooth muscle?

4. What is a motor unit? Describe the structure of a myoneural junction (motor endplate) associated with a skeletal muscle fiber.

(李晓文)

Chapter 7 Nervous Tissue

Nervous tissue, one of the four basic or primary body tissues, possesses two major cell types: nerve cells or neurons, and neuroglia or simply, glia. Neurons can generate nervous impulses in response to stimuli and transmit them along the cellular processes. Glial cells are non-impulse-conducting cells that represent the interstitial tissue which supports and protects neurons. A neuron is a highly polarized cell that consists of a soma from which the cytoplasmic processes arise. The soma also known as the cell body or perikaryon shows a prominent nucleus which is occupied mainly by enchromatin. The processes are known as the nerve fibers or neurites comprising one or more branching dendrites and often a single axon of uniform diameter. The dendrites normally conduct impulses toward the cell body, whereas axon conveys impulses away from it. The sites where nerve impulses are transmitted from a neuron to another or to an effector cells such as muscle cell or cell of a gland are called synapses.

The axon of some neurons in the central nervous system (CNS) or peripheral nervous system (PNS) is ensheathed by a layer of myelin formed by the plasmalemma of glial cells. The axons with a myelin sheath surrounding it are regarded as myelinated nerve fibers; those lacking it are unmyelinated nerve fibers (Question: Which glial cell type produces myelin in the brain and in the peripheral nerve?). The axon of a neuron terminates at different sites and the termination is called the axon terminal. The axon terminal ends either as the sensory nerve termination (free nerve endings, tactile corpuscle, lamellar corpuscle and muscle spindle) or motor nerve termination (neuromuscular junction) depending on the nature of the neuron (sensory or motor). This histological practical will emphasize on the structural organization of neurons, myelinated and unmyelinated nerve fibers. At the end of the session, you should be able to relate the microscopic structure of a neuron and different types of glial cells and nerve fibers to their functions.

【Objectives】

1. To identify and describe:

A. the microscopic structure of a neuron including the cell body, axon and dendrites.

B. the structure of a myelinated nerve fiber and differentiate it from an unmyelinated nerve fiber; also, to distinguish the difference between the myelination process in the central nervous system and that in the peripheral nervous system.

2. To understand and describe:

A. the structure of a synapse which is the site of physical and functional contacts between neurons and to define what a chemical synapse is.

B. the structure of sensory nerve termination (free nerve endings, tactile corpuscle e. g. Meissner's corpuscle, lamellar corpuscle e. g. Pacinian corpuscle, and muscle spindle) or motor nerve termination (motor end-plate or neuromusclar junction).

C. the general histological features of central nervous system, i. e. spinal cord, cerebellum, and cerebrum.

【Observation of tissue sections】

1. Neurons, Spinal cord, H & E

In a histological section, the spinal cord is organized into white matter and gray matter. The white matter is located at the peripheral zone. It does not contain any nerve cell bodies. The characteristic feature of the white matter is its closely packed nerve fibers, most of them are myelinated. These nerve fibers represent the ascending and descending axons forming the fiber tracts e. g. spinothalamic tracts, spinocerebellar tracts and corticospinal tracts in the spinal cord. In addition to the massive nerve fibers, the white matter shows various types of glial cells. (What are the types of glial cells? Review their respective functions).

The central area of the spinal cord is occupied by the gray matter containing the cell bodies of neurons, as well as the initial and terminal ends of their processes (axons and dendrites), many of them are not myelinated. The gray matter is subdivided into two main regions, the dorsal and the ventral horns. An H&E preparation showing an area of the ventral horn is illustrated (Figure 7-1). The multipolar neurons and their projecting processes are clearly evident in the ventral horn. The nucleus of the ventral horn cells (efferent neurons or motoneurons) is large and spherical, and is lightly stained because it shows mainly euchromatin (Question: What is the difference between euchromatin and heterochromatin in terms of transcription

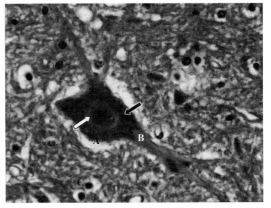

Figure 7-1   Neuron, Spinal cord, H & E
A: Cell body; B: Dendrite; C: Neuroglial cell; White arrow: Nucleus; Black arrow: Nissl body

function?). The nucleus often contains a spherical, conspicuous and darkly stained nucleolus. Question: What is the main function of the nucleolus? Note the clumps of basophilic materials in the cytoplasm termed Nissl bodies. They are identified to be the rough endoplasmic reticulum by electron microscopy. The neuropil shows a variable number of small nuclei representing the various neuroglial cell types (neuropil: area of interlacing tissue between neurons). The cytoplasm of these cells is not evident. Are you able to distinguish the axon from the dendrites?

2. Myelinated nerve fibers, Sciatic nerve, H & E

This slide has two tissue sections of the sciatic nerve: one is a longitudinal section of the nerve; the other is a transverse section. At a higher magnification in a longitudinal section of the nerve (Figure 7-2), the containing axons which are closely packed and in parallel arrays are pinkish in staining. Each axon occupies a central position; it is surrounded by a layer of myelin sheath most of which is lost during the preparation of the tissue. What is left behind as seen is a pale-staining empty looking space extending from the axon to the neurilemma. When you move your field around and adjust the focus of the tissue section, you may be able to see a few nodes of Ranvier (white arrow, Figure 7-2). The neurilemma appears as a thin membrane. In some areas, you may be able to identify the nucleus of the Schwann cells (arrowhead, Figure 7-2) in the neurilemmal sheath. Between the nerve fibers may be seen the endoneurium which contains a few fibroblasts.

A transverse section through a sciatic nerve is shown (Figure 7-3). The nerve fibers are grouped in bundles of different sizes by perineurium. The bundles are enveloped by a layer of epineurium. The latter covers the whole nerve and contains some fat cells (adipocytes) and blood vessels.

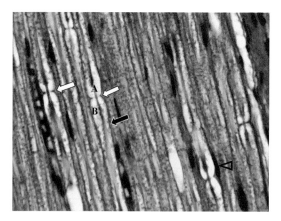

Figure 7-2   Myelinated nerve fibers (longitudinal), Sciatic nerve, H & E

A: Axon; B: Myelin sheath; White arrows: Nodes of Ranvier; Black arrow: Neurilemma; Arrowhead: Nucleus of the Schwann cell

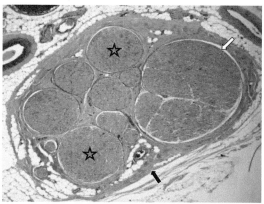

Figure 7-3   Sciatic nerve (transverse), H & E

Black arrow: Epineurium; White arrow: Perineurium; Asterisks: Nerve fiber bundles

At a higher magnification (Figure 7-4), the axon is in the center of the myelin sheath and occasionally a crescent-shaped nucleus of a Schwann cell may be seen associated with it.

3. Unmyelinated nerve fibers, Peripheal nerve, H & E

A transverse section shows several peripheral nerve fiber bundles or fasciculi containing mainly unmyelinated nerve fibers (Figure 7-5). List the differences between myelinated and unmyelinated nerve fibers. In what way does the myelin sheath facilitate the conduction of impulse along the axon?

【Demonstration slides】

1. Synapses, Spinal cord, Silver stain

Light micrograph of a neuron showing the chemical synapses which appear as brown-black knobs near or associated with the nerve cell body or dendrites called the synaptic boutons (Figure 7-6).

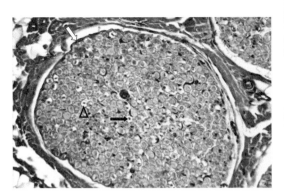

**Figure 7-4 Sciatic nerve (transverse),
H & E**

Black arrow: Axon;Arrowhead: Myelin sheath;

White arrow: Perineurium

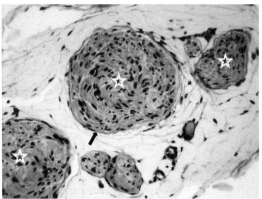

**Figure 7-5 Unmyelinated nerve fibers,
Peripheal nerve (transverse), H & E**

Black arrow: Perineurium; Asterisks:Nerve fiber
bundles

2. A multipolar neuron, Neutral carmine stain

In a histological section (Figure 7-7), a multipolar neuron has multiple dendrites, and a single axon (not shown). The cell body of the multipolar neuron is the central portion of the cell where the nucleus and perinuclear cytoplasm are located.

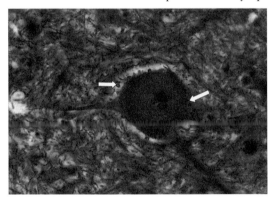

Figure 7-6 Synapses, Silver stain

White arrows: Synaptic boutons

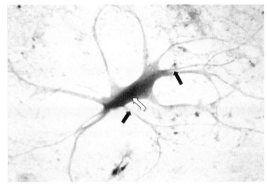

**Figure 7-7 A multipolar neuron, Neutral
carmine stain**

White arrow: Nucleus; Black arrows: Dendrites

3. Myenteric nerve plexus, Duodenum, H & E

Between the muscle layers (inner circular and outer longitudinal), you may find the myenteric nerve plexus of Auerbach containing parasympathetic postganglionic neurons (Figure 7-8). Question: How is the myenteric nerve plexus mediated by the vagus (X) nerve? What is its function?

4. Nissl body (substance), Spinal cord, Thionin stain

Identify the prominent clumps of basophilic material, Nissl substance in the cell body

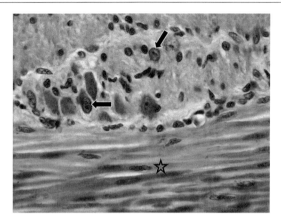

Figure 7-8　Myenteric nerve plexus, H & E
Black arrows: Neurons (parasympathetic postganglionic);
Asterisk: Smooth muscle

(Figure 7-9). Electron microscopy has revealed that the Nissl substance or body represents the rough endoplasmic reticulum (rER). Nissl body is also present in the dendrites in addition to its accumulation in the cytoplasm. It is, however, absent in the axon as well as in the funnel-shaped axon hillock from which the axon arises.

5. Neurofibrils, Spinal cord, Silver stain

The neuronal cytoskeleton contains neurofibrils in the form of dark filamentous clumps and strands coursing through the cytoplasm of the soma and extending into the processes as seen by light microscopy (Figure 7-10).

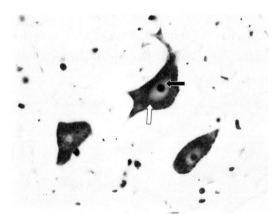

Figure 7-9　Neurons, Thionin stain
Black arrow: Nucleus; White arrow: Nissl body

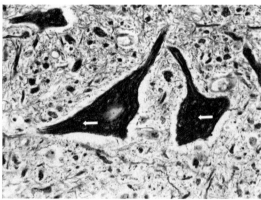

Figure 7-10　Neurons, Silver stain
White arrows: Neurofibrils

6. Myelin sheath, Osmium stain

An osmium-stained section shows the myelinated nerve fibers whose covering myelin sheath is stained black (black arrow, Figure 7-11). Note the node of Ranvier (white arrow, Figure 7-11), a region which is not covered by myelin sheath; it facilitates saltatory conduction of impulses.

7. Pacinian corpuscles, Skin, H & E

Pacinian corpuscles, located in the dermis and hypodermis, are mechanoreceptors (for detection of deep pressure sensation and vibration). Each corpuscle shows a central core (inner bulb) containing often a sensory nerve fiber with its branches and it functions as a dendrite by transmitting impulse toward the cell body (N. B. the cell body of the nerve fibers is located in the dorsal root ganglion. Note also that the sensory fiber in the corpuscle represents the peripheral process of the pseudo-unipolar neuron housed in the sensory ganglion). The outer bulb region of the Pacinian corpuscle is formed by concentrically arranged lamellae and between them may be present a variable number of epthelioid fibroblast-like cells considered by some as modified Schwann cells intermingled with collagen fibrils. The entire Pacinian corpuscle is covered by a thin layer of capsule composed of connective tissue. Pacinian corpuscles are readily recognizable in section since they resemble the cut surface of an onion (Figure 7-12).

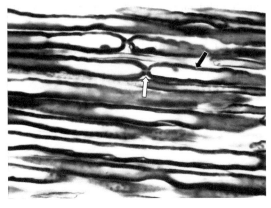

Figure 7-11　Myelinated nerve fibers, Osmium stain

Black arrow: Myelin sheath; White arrow: Node of Ranvier

8. Meissner's corpuscles, Finger tip skin, H & E

Meissner's corpuscles are tactile receptors located in dermal papillae of the skin. In a histological section (Figure 7-13), they are elongated and encapsulated. Meissner's corpuscles are commonly seen the finger tip.

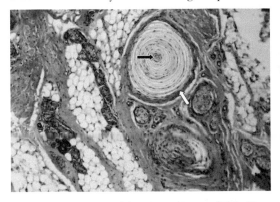

Figure 7-12　Pacinian corpuscle, H & E

Black arrow: Core; White arrow: Capsule

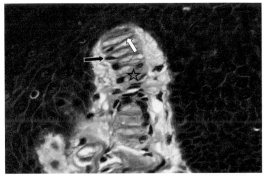

Figure 7-13　Meissner's corpuscle, H & E

Asterisk: Meissner's corpuscle; Black arrow: Nucleus of modified Schwann cell; White arrow: Nerve fiber intertwined with modified Schwann cells

9. Muscle spindle, H & E

Muscle spindle (Figure 7-14), is an encapsulated sensory receptor. Each muscle spindle is composed of 8 to 10 narrow, very small, modified muscle cells called the intrafusal fibers, surrounded by a fluid-containing periaxial space, which in turn is enclosed by the capsule. Question: What are the main functions of a muscle (neuromuscular) spindle?

10. Myoneural junction, Gold chloride stain

The image shows a myoneural junction. In the latter, when the axon reaches the vicinity of the skeletal muscle fiber, it loses its covering myelin sheath. The axon terminal gives rise to a cluster of small swellings forming the motor end-plates and abutting on the sarcolemma of the skeletal muscle fibers to which it innervates (Figure 7-15).

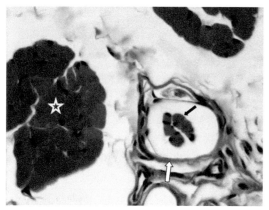

Figure 7-14 Muscle spindle, H & E

Black arrow: Intrafusal fibers; White arrow: Capsule; Asterisk: Skeletal muscle

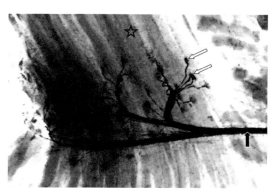

Figure 7-15 Myoneural junction, Gold chloride stain

Black arrow: Nerve fiber; White arrows: Motor end-plates; Asterisk: Skeletal muscle

11. Cerebrum, H & E

The gray matter (A, Figure 7-16) in the cerebral cortex is located at the periphery of the cerebral hemispheres and is folded into many gyri and sulci. The white matter (B, Figure 7-16) is located beneath or deep to the gray matter. The cerebral cortex (gray matter) shows six layers of neurons intermingled with glial cells (neuroglial cells). The six layers of the cortex are not clearly defined, but are nevertheless indicated as shown in Figure 7-17. Layer one of the cortex is known as the molecular layer (A, Figure 7-17), which contains numerous fibers and some scattered neuronal cell bodies. It is difficult to distinguish the neuronal soma from the neuroglial cells at this magnification. The second, external granular layer (B, Figure 7-17), is composed of small granule cells, and a large number of neuroglial cells. The third layer is known as the external pyramidal layer (C, Figure 7-17), which is the thickest layer in this section of the cerebral cortex. It consists of pyramidal cells, and some granule cells as well as numerous neuroglia interspersed among the neuronal somata and fibers. The fourth layer, the internal granular layer (D, Figure 7-17), is a relatively narrow band whose cell population consists mostly of small and a few large granule cells and

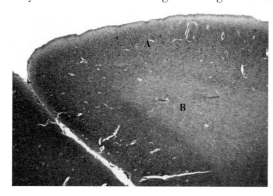

Figure 7-16 Cerebrum, H & E

A: Cerebral cortex (gray matter); B: White matter

the ever present neuroglial cells. The internal pyramidal layer (E, Figure 7-17) houses the medium and large pyramidal cells as well as the ubiquitous neuroglia, whose nuclei appear as small dots. The deepest layer of the cerebral cortex is the multiform layer (F, Figure 7-17), which contains cells of various shapes, mostly fusiform. The white matter appears very cellular, due to the presence of a large population of neuroglial cells providing support for the cell processes either emanate from or project to the cortex.

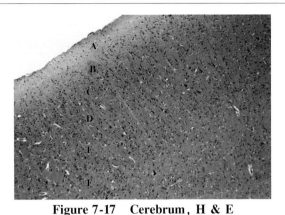

Figure 7-17　Cerebrum, H & E

A: Molecular layer; B: External granular layer; C: External pyramidal layer; D: Internal granular layer; E: Internal pyramidal layer; F: Multiform layer

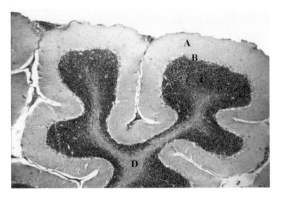

Figure 7-18　Cerebellum, H & E

A: Molecular layer; B: Purkinje cell (neuron) layer; C: Granular layer; D: White matter

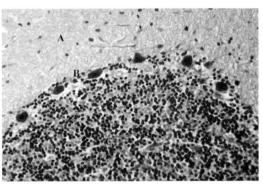

Figure 7-19　Cerebellum, H & E

A: Molecular layer; B: Purkinje cell (neuron) layer; C: Granular layer

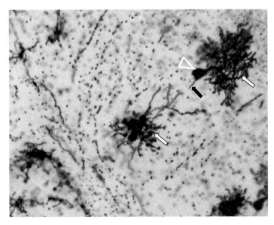

Figure 7-20　Purkinje cells (neurons), Silver stain

Arrowhead: Cell body; Black arrow: Axon; White arrows: Dendrites

12. Cerebellum, H & E

The cerebellum consists of a core of white matter and the superficially located gray matter (Figure 7-18). The gray matter is subdivided into three distinct layers: the outer molecular layer, a middle Purkinje cell layer, and the inner granular layer (Figure 7-18, Figure 7-19).

13. Purkinje cells (neurons), Silver stain

The Purkinje cells (Figure 7-20) or neurons of the cerebellar cortex are multipolar neurons, whose cell body is pear-shaped bearing large, branching dendrites that enter the molecular layer, and a single axon that projects from the base of the cell into the granular layer and thence to the deep cerebellar nuclei.

【Questions and topics for discussion and integration】

1. Describe the histological features of a typical neuron in the central nervous system (brain or spinal cord).

2. What are the types of neuroglial cells in the brain? Describe the microscopic features of each of them and mention briefly their functions.

3. Describe the structure of a sensory ganglion (dorsal root ganglion) as seen under the light microscope. Name two sites in the peripheral tissues where the processes of sensory neurons terminate.

4. Describe the histological features of a peripheral nerve, e. g. sciatic nerve, as seen under the light microscope.

5. Name the peripheral sensory receptors in the skin. Describe their structure and functions.

6. Describe the electron microscopic structure of a chemical synapse between two neurons.

7. What are the main functions of the cerebellum?

(李娟娟)

Chapter 8   Integument

The integument, composed of skin and its appendages including the sweat glands, sebaceous glands, hair, and nails, is the largest organ of the body. Skin serves as a protective barrier against injury, infectious pathogens, and ultraviolet radiation, but also assists in body temperature regulation, vitamin D synthesis, ion excretion, and sensory reception. The following are the learning objectives for this histological practical class.

【Objectives】

1. To identify and describe the basic structure of skin (thin and thick): epidermis and dermis.

2. To understand and describe the various derivatives of skin: sweat glands, sebaceous glands, arrector pili muscle, and hair.

3. To understand and describe the structure of hypodermis (subcutaneous tissue or superficial fascia).

【Observation of tissue sections】

1. Thick skin, Fingertip skin, H & E

This is a section of thick skin from the finger. It is made up of a superficial layer of epidermis and an underlying deeper layer of dermis (Figure 8-1). The epidermis is the epithelial layer. Question: What type of epithelium forms the epidermis? The underlying dermis is subdivided into two regions, a papillary layer, composed of the loose connective tissue in the dermal papilla, and in the deeper region, the reticular layer which is composed of dense connective tissue. The fatty connective tissue layer, known as the hypodermis but not a part of the skin, lies beneath the dermis. In the dermis or hypodermis, identify the Pacinian corpuscles. Meissner's corpuscles may be found in the dermal papillae.

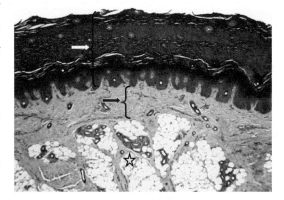

Figure 8-1   Thick skin, Fingertip skin, H & E
White arrow: Epidermis; Black arrow: Dermis; Asterisk: Hypodermis

At a higher magnification, the epidermis consists of the various layers, namely, the stratum basale (germinativum), stratum spinosum, stratum granulosum, stratum lucidum and stratum corneum (Figure 8-2). Identify the various layers of the epidermis from the basal to apical surface. In the dermis, or hypodermis, look for sweat glands and identify the secretory portion and duct of the glands (Figure 8-3). Question: What is the innervation of the sweat glands?

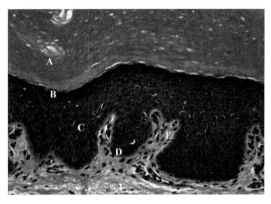

Figure 8-2 Thick skin, Fingertip skin, H & E

A: Stratum corneum; B: Stratum granulosum; C: Stratum spinosum; D: Stratum basale; E: Papillary layer; F: Reticular layer

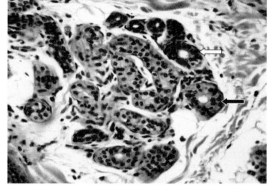

Figure 8-3 Sweat glands, H & E

White arrow: Duct; Black arrow: Secretory portion

2. Thin skin, Scalp, H & E

This is a section of thin skin from the scalp. Thin skin is composed of a very slender layer of epidermis and the underlying dermis (Figure 8-4). Can you identify the adipose subcutaneous tissue? Hair follicles, arrector pili muscle and sebaceous glands are absent in the thick skin. They are however common features of the thin skin. Most part of the hair follicle is embedded beneath the skin in the superficial fascia. Examine the hair follicle, whose expanded bulb shows the connective tissue papilla (Figure 8-5). Sebaceous glands secrete their sebum into the lumen of the hair follicle (Figure 8-6). Blockage of the gland secretion may result in infection causing pimples or ACNE. Smooth muscle bundles (arrector pili muscle) cradle these glands and they extend from the hair follicle to the papillary layer of the dermis (Figure 8-6). Contraction of this muscle causes "goose pimples". Identify a hair follicle, sebaceous gland and its associated arrector pili muscle.

【Demonstration slide】

Melanocytes, H & E

Melanocytes derived from neural crest cells, are responsible for the manufacture of melanin, which is synthesized on specialized organelles called melanosomes. They are interspersed among the keratinocytes in the stratum basale and are also present in hair follicles. They possess long thin cytoplasmic processes that extend into the intercellular spaces between cells of the stratum spinosum. This tissue section shows melanin granules which are distributed in the keratinocytes of the stratum basale and stratum spinosum (Figure 8-7).

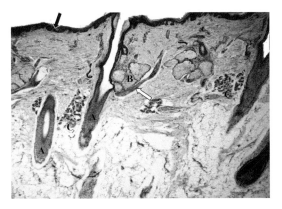

Figure 8-4   Thin skin, Scalp, H & E

A: Hair follicles; B: Sebaceous glands; C: Sweat glands; White arrow: Arrector pili muscle; Black arrow: Epidermis

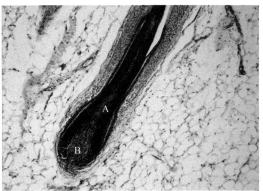

Figure 8-5   Hair follicle, H & E

A: Hair bulb; B: Hair papilla

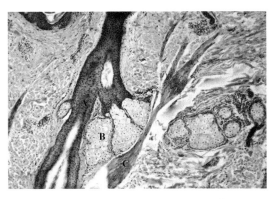

Figure 8-6   Skin derivatives, H & E

A: Hair follicle; B: Sebaceous gland; C: Arrector pili muscle

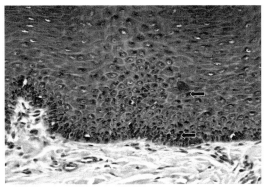

Figure 8-7   Melanocytes, H & E

Black arrows: Melanin granules

【Questions and topics for discussion and integration】

1. Describe the histology of the thin skin. Correlate this with its functions.

2. Describe the histology of the skin at the finger tip. What are the layers of the epidermis?

3. Describe the histology of the skin of the sole.

4. Highlight the histological differences between the thin and thick skin.

(周　琳)

Chapter 9　Cardiovascular System

The cardiovascular system consists of the heart and closed vessels through which blood circulates in the body. Heart pumps the blood to the arteries. Arteries branch repeatedly, and have smaller diameters as they course toward the periphery. The arteries are classified into three types, namely, elastic arteries, muscular arteries (distributing arteries or medium-sized arteries)and arterioles, based on the vascular size and the characteristic features of the walls, such as the tunica media. The muscular arteries deliver blood to capillaries, which are the thinnest vessels and are the sites of exchange of gases, nutrients and other substances occurring between the blood and tissues. Blood is returned to the heart via medium-sized and large veins, e. g. inferior vena cava. The walls of blood vessels whose diameters are larger than the capillary have three distinct layers, or tunics: inner tunica intima, middle tunica media, and outer tunica adventitia.

【Objectives】

1. To identify and describe:

A. the histological features of the heart wall: endocardium, myocardium, epicardium, and Purkinje fibers.

B. the histological structure of different layers of arteries: tunica intima, tunica media, tunica adventitia, internal and external elastic lamina.

C. the histological differences between the elastic and muscular arteries.

2. To understand and describe the common features of veins; also, to differentiate these from those in the arteries.

3. To understand and describe the main histological structure of the capillaries (fenestrated [discontinuous] and non-fenestrated [continuous] capillaries).

【Observation of tissue sections】

1. Heart, H & E

The heart is a hollow muscular organ. Its wall consists of three layers: endocardium, myocardium and epicardium (Figure 9-1, Figure 9-2). The innermost layer endocardium is composed of an endothelium, a type of simple squamous epithelium, and the underlying connective tissue, subendothelial layer (Figure 9-3). Locate the bundles of Purkinje fibers (specialized cardiac muscle fibers) in the subendothelial region and note their distinguishing features. They are larger than the normal myocardial cells (myocytes). Note that the nucleus of the Purkinje fibers is centrally placed. The region where the Purkinje fibers are located is called the subendocardial layer. The myocardium is the thickest layer in the heart wall; it consists mostly of cardiac muscle cells or fibers. The bundles of muscle fibers run in different directions. Loose connective tissue lies between the muscle fibers with abundant capillaries and occasionally may be present some lymphatic vessels (Figure 9-3, Figure 9-4). The outer layer is the epicardium (Figure 9-4) which has two layers: the deeper loose, fatty connective tissue and external to this, the mesothelium (Figure 9-4), a single layer of flattened epithelial cells.

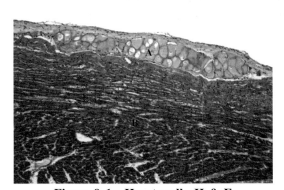

Figure 9-1   Heart wall, H & E

A: Endocardium; B: Myocardium

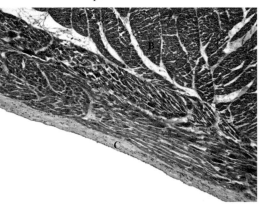

Figure 9-2   Heart wall, H & E

B: Myocardium; C: Epicardium

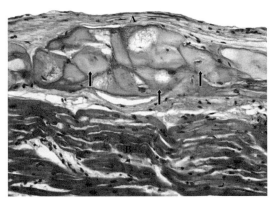

Figure 9-3   Heart wall, H & E

A: Endocardium; B: Myocardium; Black arrows:
Purkinje fibers

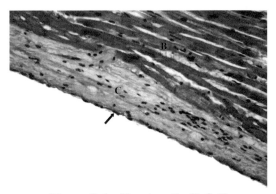

Figure 9-4   Heart wall, H & E

B: Myocardium; C: Epicardium; Black arrow:
Mesothelium

2. Elastic artery, H & E

The elastic arteries (or large arteries) conduct blood from the heart to muscular arteries. Note the three basic layers of the arterial wall (Figure 9-5): tunica intima, tunica media and tunica adventitia.

The tunica media is the most prominentlayer of the three (tunica intima, media and adventitia) in the arterial wall (Figure 9-6, Figure 9-7). It consists of abundant elastic fibers organized as 40 ~ 70 concentric, fenestrated elastic laminae.

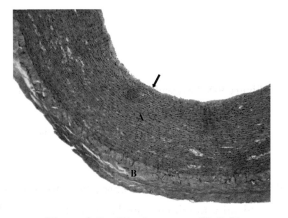

Figure 9-5   Elastic artery, H & E

Black arrow: Tunica intima; A: Tunica media; B: Tunica
adventitia

Between the elastic laminae are present the collagen fibers admixed with smooth muscle cells (Figure 9-6, Figure 9-7). The elastic laminae are stained bright pink. There is no distinct internal or external lamina; hence, the three layers of the arterial wall can not be clearly distinguished. In the adventitia (Figure 9-7), note the presence of small blood vessels (vasa vasorum) supplying the vessel wall, and fat cells. Question: What cells synthesize the elastic fibers or elastic lamina?

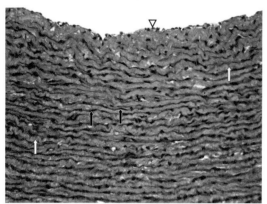 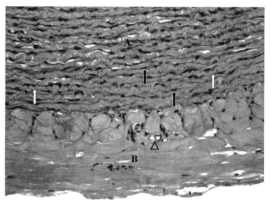

Figure 9-6 Elastic artery, H & E

A: Tunica media; Arrowhead: Endothelium; White arrows: Elastic lamina; Black arrows: Smooth muscle cells

Figure 9-7 Elastic artery, H & E

A: Tunica media; B: Tunica adventitia; White arrows: Elastic lamina; Black arrows: Smooth muscle cells; Arrowhead: Small blood vessel (vasa vasorum)

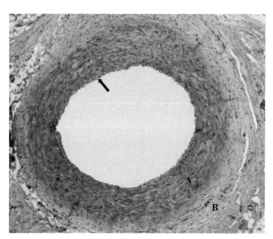

Figure 9-8 Muscular artery (medium-sized artery), H & E

Black arrow: Tunica intima; A: Tunica media; B: Tunica adventitia

3. Muscular arteries and veins, H & E

A muscular artery (distributing or medium-sized artery) and its accomp-anying medium-sized vein are seen (Figure 9-8, Figure 9-9). The wall of both vessels has three layers: the tunica intima, tunica media and tunica adventitia. First, distinguish the artery from the vein. The artery has a thicker and more regular tunica media than the vein. In histological preparations they more often retain their round profiles when cut in cross section. Veins tend to appear "collapsed" or flattened under the same circumstances. In addition, the tunica media of vein is much thinner than in artery; in contrast, the adventitia is much thicker than that of an artery.

Identify the three main layers of the artery, and also the two elastic laminae (Figure 9-10). The tunica intima is the thinnest of the three layers. Smooth muscle dominates the tunica media. Between the smooth muscle layers in the tunica media are a variable number of elastic fibers intermingled with collagen fibers. The tunica adventitia is loose connective tissue. A distinct internal elastic lamina is seen at the border between the intima and media, and an external elastic lamina at the interface between the media and the adventitia. The elastic laminae are bright refractive wave-like bands. The internal and external elastic laminae are poorly developed in the vein, thus the borders between the three layers in its wall are less evident (Figure 9-11). Question: What is the innervation of the smooth muscle fibers in the blood vessel wall?

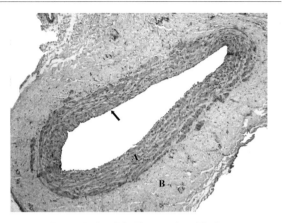

Figure 9-9   Medium vein, H & E
Black arrow: Tunica intima; A: Tunica media;
B: Tunica adventitia

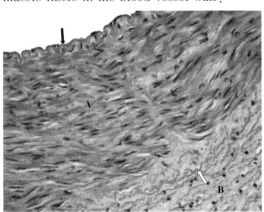

Figure 9-10   Muscular artery (medium sized artery) , H & E
A: Tunica media; B: Tunica adventitia; Black arrow: Internal elastic lamina; White arrow: External elastic lamina

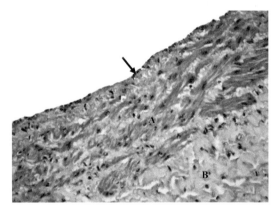

Figure 9-11   Medium vein, H & E
Black arrow: Tunica intima; A: Tunica media;
B: Tunica adventitia

Muscular arteries (A, Figure 9-12) of a smaller caliber have a thicker wall and smaller lumen comparing with the accompanying small veins (B, Figure 9-12). The tunica media is composed of smooth muscle cells and, hence, the vessel is classified as the muscular artery. The internal elastic lamina is extremely thin or absent in arteries that are of the smaller caliber. How does the muscular artery differ from its companion vein in histology?

4. Arterioles and venules, capillaries, H & E

Look for arterioles, venules and capillaries embedded in the connective tissue between the main vessels. Arteriole has a small lumen and its tunica media is composed of only 1 ~ 2 layers of small muscle cells (Figure 9-13). Capillaries are simple tubes with a very thin wall, consisting of an endothelium with only 2 ~ 3 endothelial cells (Figure 9-13). The nucleus is small and flattened.

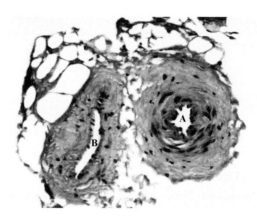

Figure 9-12 Muscular artery (small-sized artery) and small vein, H & E

A:Small-sized artery; B: Small vein

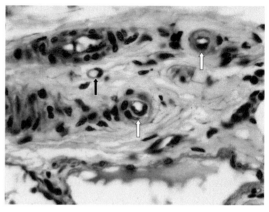

Figure 9-13 Arteriole and capillary, H & E

White arrows: Arterioles; Black arrow: Capillary

Do a self-assessment and to make sure that you are able to distinguish the arteries/arterioles from the veins/venules.

Many veins with a diameter more than 2 mm, especially veins in the limbs, are provided with semilunar folds of the tunica intima projecting into the lumen, which are termed the valves of vein (Figure 9-14). They usually occur in pairs, whose function is to aid the flow of blood toward the heart and prevent the flow in the reverse direction.

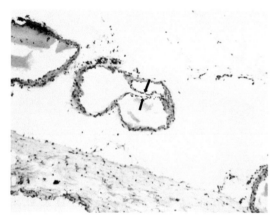

Figure 9-14 Valve of vein, H & E

Black arrows: Valves of vein

【Demonstration slides】

1. Elastic artery, Elastic stain

The thick tunica media shows the distinct multilayered and wavy elastic laminae(Figure 9-15).

2. Muscular artery,Special stain

The staining is specifically for elastic fibers(Figure 9-16). The elastic fibers are stained in deep purple, while the smooth muscle cells are in red. The internal elastic lamina is readily identifiable which appears as a continuous and conspicuous wavy line in comparison with the external elastic lamina.

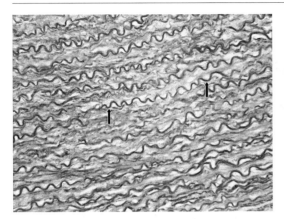

Figure 9-15　Elastic artery, Elastic stain

Black arrows: Elastic laminae

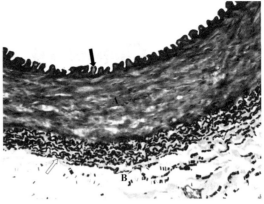

Figure 9-16　Muscular artery, Special stain

A: Tunica media; B: Tunica adventitia; Black arrow: Internal elastic lamina; White arrow: External elastic lamina

【Questions and topics for discussion and integration】

1. What are the layers of tissue forming the walls of the heart and major blood vessels? Do blood capillaries show similar tissue layers?

2. Describe the histology of the Purkinje fibers in the conducting system of the heart. How do they differ from the main cardiac muscle fibers?

3. Describe the differences between the two major types of blood capillaries: fenestrated (discontinuous) and non-fenestrated (continuous). Where are they distributed?

4. Describe the histology of a muscular artery. Highlight its major differences from a vein.

5. Give an account of the histology of the major elastic artery and give two representative examples of elastic arteries.

(袁　云)

Chapter 10   Immune System

The immune system consists of groups of immune molecules (immunoglobulin), cells, tissues and organs, which defend the body against invading microorganisms and other harmful antigenic substances, and monitor the changes within the body. Lymphatic organs are classified in functional terms as primary and secondary lymphatic organs. Lymphocytes migrate from the primary (or central) organs e. g. thymus and bone marrow to the blood and secondary (or peripheral) organs, e. g. spleen, lymph nodes and tonsils, where they proliferate, complete their differentiation and execute their immune functions.

【Objectives】

1. To identify and describe:

A. the histological features of the lymph node: capsule, cortex (cortical sinus, lymphatic nodules, thymus-dependent region), medulla (medullary cords and medullary sinuses).

B. the histological features of the spleen: capsule, red pulp (splenic cords and splenic sinuses), white pulp (lymphatic nodules and periarterial lymphatic sheaths).

C. the histological features of the thymus: capsule, cortex and medulla (thymic or Hassall's corpuscles).

2. To understand and describe the main histological features of the palatine tonsil.

【Observation of tissue sections】

1. Lymph node, H & E

Examine the slide with the naked eye. In Figure 10-1 and Figure 10-2, identify the medulla (paler central area) and the cortex (periphery with lymphatic nodules). First, under low power objective lens, identify the connective tissue capsule surrounding the entire mass of the lymphatic tissue (Figure 10-3). Trabeculae (pinkish fibrous bundles) are seen extending from the capsule into the parenchyma of the lymph node to form part of the supporting stroma. Some adipose tissue is present around the lymph node. The hilum (white arrow, Figure 10-1) may be identified in some slides. The hilum or hilus is the site where efferent lymphatic vessel draining the lymph fluid leaves the lymph node.

The darkly stained cortex immediately

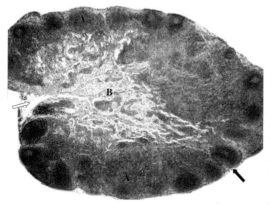

Figure 10-1   Lymph node, H & E
A: Cortex; B: Medulla; Black arrow: Capsule; White arrow: Hilum

beneath the capsule consists of lymphatic nodules (Figure 10-3) , paracortex and cortical sinuses. Identify the subcapsular sinus, a narrow channel just beneath the capsule, and trabecular sinuses that accompany the trabeculae. B lymphocytes (B cells) predominate in the lymphatic nodules, while T lymphocytes (T cells) are distributed mainly in the paracortex or thymus-dependent region (zone) (Figure 10-3). Examine one of the lymphatic nodules. Can
you recognize the germinal centre? Are there any cells undergoing mitosis?

The medulla is a pale-staining area that varies in width and abuts the hilum (Figure 10-
4, Figure 10-5). It is characterized by the presence of the medullary cords (loosely arranged
lymphatic tissue) separated by medullary sinuses (lymphatic channels). Sectional profiles of
irregularly arranged trabecula also occupy the medulla.

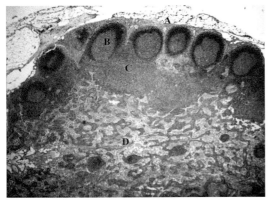

Figure 10-2   Lymph node, H & E
A: Capsule; B: Lymphatic nodule; C: Paracortex;
D: Medulla

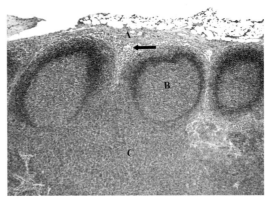

Figure 10-3   Lymph node, H & E
A: Capsule; B: Lymphatic nodule; C: Paracortex;
Black arrow: Cortical sinus

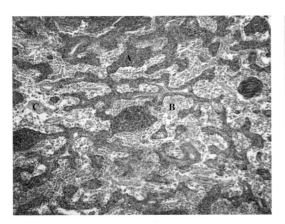

Figure 10-4   Lymph node, H & E
A: Medullary cords; B: Medullary sinuses;
C: Trabecula

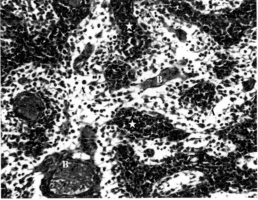

Figure 10-5   Lymph node, H & E
Asterisk: Medullary cords; A: Medullary sinuses;
B: Trabecula (contains a vein filled with red blood
cells)

2. Spleen, H & E

Examine the slide first with the naked eye. Identify the red pulp (reddish violet areas), and the white pulp (scattered deep blue spherical areas). At low power, what are the distinguishing histological features between the spleen and the lymph node? The spleen (Figure 10-6) is covered by a thick connective tissue capsule which has a larger component of elastic fibers, smooth muscle cells and a covering layer of mesothelium. Trabecula from the capsule extends into the splenic parenchyma. Unlike other lymphoid organs, the spleen does not have a cortex or a medulla; instead, it is made up of splenic pulps termed the white pulp and red pulp, based on the coloring as seen in a fresh tissue. The white pulp appears as grayish white due to the islands of lymphoid tissue, whereas the red pulp is so named because of its contents of abundant erythrocytes.

The white pulp (Figure 10-7) consists of lymphatic tissue that forms the periarterial (or periarteriolar) lymphatic sheath (PALS) surrounding the central artery (black arrow, Figure 10-7) and the lymphatic nodules. T cells are found mainly in PALS around the central artery. Lymphatic nodules lie in the more peripheral white pulp relative to the arteries. As in the lymph node, B cells aggregate in the primary lymphatic nodule or secondary nodule with a germinal center. Central arteries may be seen traversing the lymphatic nodules. Surrounding the white pulp is a shell of sparsely cellular lymphatic tissue—the marginal zone, which is not easily defined.

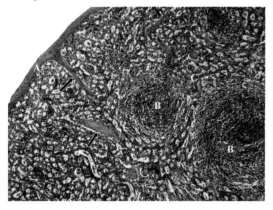

Figure 10-6   Spleen, H & E

A: Capsule; B: White pulp; C: Red pulp; Black arrow:Trabecula

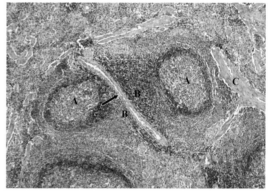

Figure 10-7   Spleen, H & E

A:Lymphatic nodules (Malpighian corpuscles); B: Periarterial lymphatic sheaths; C: Trabecula; Black arrow: Central artery

The tissue spaces between the white pulps are occupied by the red pulp (Figure 10-8), which constitutes mostly of the splenic cords and between them the sinuses. The splenic cords consist of a cellular network of reticular cells in contact with one another. The network contains lymphocytes, plasma cells, numerous macrophages and extravasated erythrocytes. The splenic sinuses are thin-walled venous sinusoids engorged with erythrocytes.

3. Thymus, H & E

Examine the thymus under the low power and locate the capsule, septa and lobules (Figure 10-9). Each lobule has a peripheral cortex and central medulla (Figure 10-10). The cortex appears darker as it contains densely packed lymphocytes. Scattered throughout the medulla are concentrically arranged cellular aggregates known as the thymic or Hassall's corpuscles. At a higher magnification (Figure 10-11), Hassall's corpuscles are made up of epithelial reticular cells in a spherical arrangement. Question: What are the functions of the epithelial reticular cells?

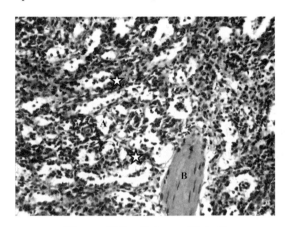

Figure 10-8　Spleen, H & E

A: Splenic sinuses; B: Trabecula; Asterisks:
Splenic cords (Cords of Billroth)

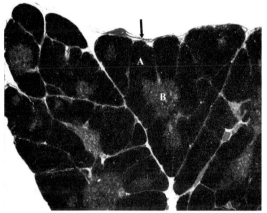

Figure 10-9　Thymus, H & E

A: Cortex; B: Medulla; Black arrow: Capsule

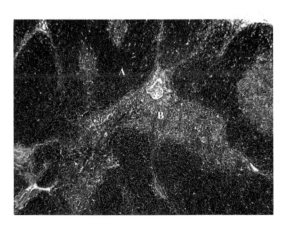

Figure 10-10　Thymus, H & E

A: Cortex; B: Medulla

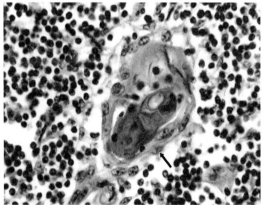

Figure 10-11　Thymus, H & E

Black arrow: Hassall's corpuscle with epithelial
reticular cells

【Demonstration slides】

Palatine tonsil, H & E

Note the stratified squamous epithelium lining the tonsillar surface (facing the oropharynx) dips into the underlying tissue in numerous places to form the tonsillar crypts. Numerous lymphatic nodules with a germinal center are present deep to the epithelial surface (Figure 10-12).

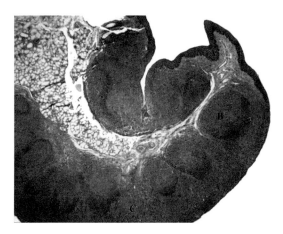

Figure 10-12   Palatine tonsil, H & E

A: Stratified squamous epithelium; B: Lymphatic nodule; C: Diffuse lymphatic tissue

【Questions and topics for discussion and integration】

1. Correlate the histology of a lymph node with its functions.

2. Describe the histology of the thymus of a child. Define the blood-thymus barrier. What is its functional significance?

3. What are the functions of the spleen? Describe its histology and the blood circulation through this organ. Compare the histological differences between the lymph node and the spleen.

4. What are the differences between the white pulp and red pulp in the spleen?

5. What are tonsils and where are they located? Describe the main histological features of the palatine tonsil. What is "tonsillitis" and what cellular activities or functions may be enhanced in this process?

(杨 力)

Chapter 11　Eye

The eye is a special sensory organ, consisting of the eyeball and associated structures including eyelids, extraocular muscles, conjunctiva and lacrimal apparatus. As the eyeball is the core structure of the eye, we will focus on its wall and its contents. The eye wall has three concentric layers: the outermost protective fibrous layer, middle vascular and pigmented layer, and the innermost layer termed the retina. The fibrous layer, also called the tunica fibrosa, consists of dense connective tissue; it includes the cornea and sclera. The junction of cornea and sclera or corneoscleral junction is called limbus. The middle vascular layer or tunica vasculosa consists of loose connective tissue. This comprises the iris, ciliary body/processes and choroid. The innermost layer or retina is mainly composed of nervous tissue. The contents of the eye, including the aqueous humor, lens and vitreous, as well as the cornea represent the refractive media of the eye. These transmit in succession the light source from the external world to the retina and thence to the brain.

【Objectives】

1. To identify and describe the light microscopic structure of cornea and retina.
2. To describe the chief histological features of the eye wall.
3. To understand the contents of the eye: lens, aqueous humor and vitreous body.

【Observation of tissue sections】

Eye wall, H & E

The eye wall is divided into three layers: tunica fibrosa, tunica vasculosa and retina. The outermost tunica fibrosa is made up of the sclera and the cornea. The opaque and whitish sclera covers the posterior five-sixths of the eyeball, whereas the colorless, transparent cornea covers the anterior one-sixth of the eyeball. Here are the general arrangement and features of the eye wall: the outermost layer is the sclera, the middle layer is choroid, and the innermost layer is the retina. Figure 11-1 shows the corneoscleral junction, also called limbus, which is the junction of the sclera with the cornea. It is an important landmark because it is situated over the trabecular meshwork and the canal of Schlemm. It is to be noted that this plays an important role in draining the aqueous humor from the anterior chamber of the eye and into the venous circulation. Cornea and sclera belong to the tunica fibrosa. Iris and ciliary body belong to the tunica vasculosa. The trabecular meshwork and the canal of Schlemm may be seen in an enlarged image (Figure 11-2). The angle formed by the iris and the corneal (limbus) is the anterior chamber angle.

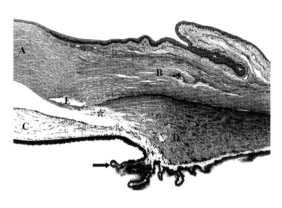

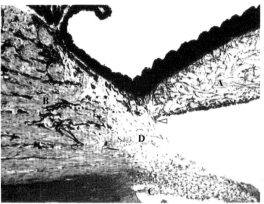

Figure 11-1 Eye wall, H & E

A: Cornea; B: Sclera; C: Iris; D: Ciliary body; E: Canal of Schlemm; Asterisk: Trabecular meshwork; Black arrow: Ciliary process

Figure 11-2 Eye wall, H & E

A: Iris; B: Ciliary body; C: Canal of Schlemm; D: Trabecular meshwork; Arrowhead: Anterior chamber angle

Cornea is a transparent and avascular fibrous tunic (Figure 11-3). Being most anteriorly placed, it helps to direct the light rays entering the eye. It is thicker than the sclera and is composed of five histologically distinct layers: corneal epithelium, anterior limiting lamina (also called Bowman's membrane), corneal stroma, posterior limiting lamina (also called Descemet's membrane), corneal endothelium. The cornea is lined by stratified squamous epithelium consisting of four to six layers of flattened cells and is about 50 mm in thickness. It has a remarkable capacity for regeneration. The cornea is avascular, of which and its state of relative dehydration give its transparency. Also, the lack of keratinization and the uniform thickness of the epithelium contribute to the transparency of the cornea which is important for light transmission. The cell surface is not entirely smooth; instead, many small microvilli appear to project from it, and they serve to anchor the vitally important tear film. Bowman's membrane is the thick basement membrane at the interface between the anterior corneal epithelium and the corneal stroma which shows mainly type I collagen fibrils. Descemet's membrane is the distinct layer of basement membrane of the posterior epithelium. It shows primarily of type VIII collagen, a relatively rare collagen type. The epithelial cells are held together by tight junctions which control the movement of water, ions, and metabolites between the stroma and the aqueous humor, the source of nutrition for the corneal stroma. Keratocytes are extremely flattened fibroblasts that produce and maintain the stroma. Corneal endothelium is a single layer of squamous cells; it functions in the regulation of water in the stroma. The primary task of corneal endothelium is to pump the excess fluid out of the stroma and, therefore, is critical for keeping the cornea clear. In the event that the endothelium is damaged, the ensuing corneal swelling due to fluid retention within the stroma may result in loss of its transparency.

The whitish sclera is composed of mainly type I collagen fibers intermingled with elastic fibers; it is nearly devoid of blood vessels. It is therefore an opaque, fibrous, and protective outer structure which provides attachment surfaces for extra-ocular muscles.

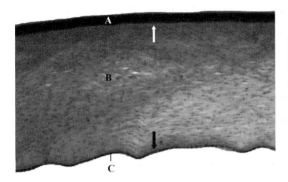

Figure 11-3   Cornea, H & E

A: Corneal epithelium; B: Corneal stroma; C: Corneal endothelium; White arrow: Anterior limiting lamina; Black arrow: Posterior limiting lamina

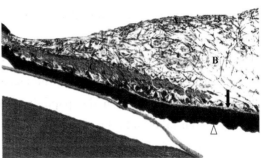

Figure 11-4   Iris, H & E

A: Anterior border layer; B: Iris stroma; C: Constrictor pupillae muscle; Black arrow: Dilator pupillae muscle; Arrowhead: Pigment epithelium

The vascular layer or tunica vasculosa consists of the iris, ciliary body and choroid. The iris (Figure 11-4) which is the anterior most extension of the choroid, lies between the posterior and anterior chambers of the eye. It completely covers the lens except at the pupil. The anterior surface of the iris (anterior border layer) consists of a discontinuous layer of fibroblasts and melanocytes. Beneath it is a thick layer of loose connective tissue, called the iris stroma, which contains some fibers, cells (fibroblasts and melanocytes) and blood vessels. The posterior surface of the iris is covered by two layers of heavily pigmented epithelial cells, which are the anterior iridial epithelium (anterior pigment epithelium) and the posterior iridial epithelium (posterior pigment epithelium). The iris has two important smooth muscles regulating the size of the pupil: dilator pupillae muscle and sphincter pupillae muscle. The dilator pupillae muscle which is supplied by the sympathetic fibers dilates the pupil. (Note that the postganglionic sympathetic neurons are located in the superior sympathetic ganglion in the neck). The sphincter pupillae muscle fibers encircling the pupil are supplied by the parasympathetic fibers (Note that the postganglionic parasympathetic neurons are located in the ciliary ganglion; the preganglionic parasympathetic neurons are located in the Edinger-Westphal nucleus in the mid-brain). Contraction of the sphincter pupillae muscle constricts the diameter of the pupil. The diameter of the pupil changes inversely with the amount of light entering it. Question: What is pupillary reflex?

The ciliary body is located between the iris and choroid. It lies internal to the anterior margin of the sclera. It is wedge-shaped in a sagittal section of the eyeball at low magnification (D, Figure 11-1). The transition between the cornea and sclera is termed the limbus. This is an important landmark for eye surgery procedures. The surface of the anterior portion of the ciliary body (ciliary process) has zonular fibers attached to it and is in contact with the aqueous humor. The junction between the ciliary body and the choroid is called ora serrata.

The ciliary body has ciliary muscle, ciliary stroma and ciliary epithelium. The ciliary muscle fibers are arranged into three orientations: longitudinal (meridional), radial and circular. Contraction and relaxation of ciliary muscles alter the shape (curvature) of lens for eye accommodation for near and distant vision. Ciliary muscles are innervated by the parasympathetic nerve fibers of the oculomotor nerve. The ciliary stroma contains connective tissue rich in blood vessels and pigment cells.

Aqueous humor is produced in the posterior chamber by the epithelium lining the ciliary processes. It flows through the pupil from the posterior chamber to the anterior chamber, where it is absorbed into the trabecular meshwork. From the latter, the aqueous humor diffuses into the canal of Schlemm and then enters the venous circulation. Blockage of the canal of Schlemm or the aqueous humor drainage system may result in increase in intraocular pressure termed glaucoma which may affect the peripheral vision or total blindness.

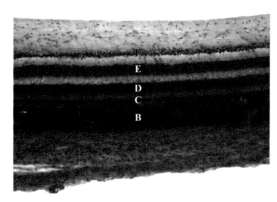

Figure 11-5 Retina, H & E

A: Sclera; B: Choroid; C: Pigment epithelium; D: Photoreceptor cell layer; E: Bipolar cell layer; F: Ganglion cell layer

The retina lies inner to the choroid which can be divided into the non-neural and the neural (visual) part bearing the photoreceptors (Figure 11-5). The neural retina is composed of four main cell layers: pigment epithelium, photoreceptor cell layer, bipolar cell (neuron) layer and ganglion cell layer.

The pigment epithelium which is rich in melanin granules forms the outermost layer of the retina. It is mainly protective in function.

The photoreptor cell layer consists of two types of photoreceptor cells, known as rod cells and cone cells. Rod and cone cells are both photoreceptor neurons. They bear some resemblances in structure and both have: a synaptic region, a nuclear region, inner segments and outer segments. There are numerous synaptic vesicles in the synaptic regions, where the photoreceptors synapse with the dendrites of the bipolar neurons. The rod cells are numerous in the peripheral retina, whereas none in the fovea. The synaptic region is spherule; it forms synaptic contacts with the dendrites of the bipolar neurons. Rods are specialized for vision in dim light. The cone photoreceptors are present in both the center and periphery of the retina but are most highly concentrated in the macula. They also form synaptic contacts with dendrites of bipolar neurons. Cones are specialized for fine visual acuity and color vision.

The bipolar neurons interlink between the photoreceptors and ganglion cells. The ganglion cells are multipolar neurons with long axons. The axons from the ganglion cells form the optic nerve whose containing fibers project to the lateral geniculate body in the thalamus, and then to the primary visual cortex localized in the occipital lobe of the cerebrum.

The papilla of the optic nerve (also called optic disk) located on the posterior wall of the eyeball, is the exit site of the optic nerve and its fibers (axons of ganglion cells). Because it is devoid of photoreceptor cells, it is insensitive to light and is therefore called the "blind spot" (Figure 11-6). Approximately 2. 5 mm lateral to the papilla of optic nerve is a yellow-pigmented zone in the retinal wall called the macula lutea (yellow spot). The central depression in the macular lutea is called the fovea centralis, where it is specialized for discrimination of details and color vision (Figure 11-7).

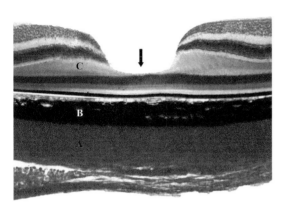

Figure 11-6   Macula lutea, H & E
A: Sclera; B: Choroid; C: Retina; Black arrow:
Fovea centralis

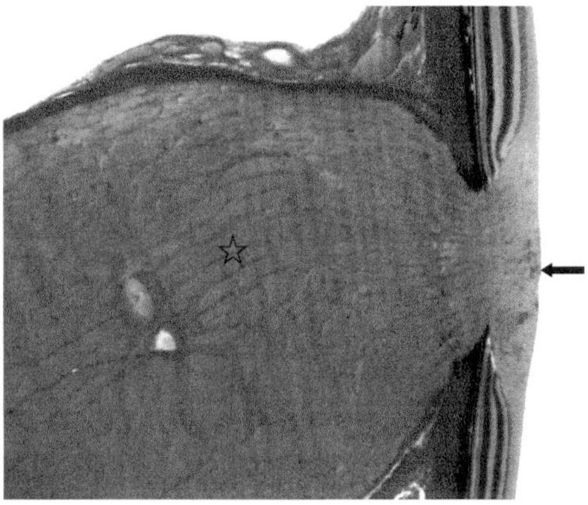

Figure 11-7   Papilla of optic nerve, H & E
Black arrow: Papilla of optic nerve; Asterisk:
Optic nerve

【Questions and clinical points for discussion and integration】

1. Describe the histological features of the cornea, iris and ciliary body. Briefly mention the innervation to each of these regions?

2. Give an account of the passage of light (light path) from the external source to the brain.

3. What are the layers of the visual (neural) retina?

4. Define the following: cataract, glaucoma, retinal tear/detachment, vitreous floaters. Explain the histological or physiological basis for the cause of each of them.

5. Describe the production, circulation and function of aqueous humor.

6. What is "accommodation of eye"? Which muscles and nerves are involved in this process?

7. How is the pupil size controlled? Name the muscles and nerves that are involved in this process.

8. Based on your knowledge in neuroanatomy, review and discuss the following: corneal reflex and pupillary reflex.

(郭小兵)

Chapter 12　Digestive Tract

The digestive or alimentary tract is a muscular tube extending from the oral cavity to the anus. The tube is structurally modified at different regions in adaptation for specific functions including digestion, secretion and absorption. The basic pattern in terms of histological organization, however, is applicable throughout the digestive tract. With the exception of the oral cavity and the pharynx, the wall of the digestive tract is made up of four principal layers: the mucosa, submucosa, muscularis externa and serosa or adventitia.

【Objectives】

1. To identify and describe:

A. the general histological structure of the digestive tract and relate this to its functions.

B. the microscopic features of the esophagus, stomach, small intestine (duodenum, jejunum, ileum) and highlight their major histological differences.

2. To understand and describe the main histological structure of the colon, appendix and rectum.

【Observation of tissue sections】

1. Esophagus, H & E

Under the low power, identify the four typical layers of the esophagus, namely, mucosa (epithelium, lamina propria and muscularis mucosa), submucosa, muscularis externa and adventitia (Figure 12-1). The esophageal mucosa is covered by a layer of nonkeratinized stratified squamous epithelium, allowing constant wear and tear because of passage of solid foods. Beneath the epithelium is a supporting layer of lamina propria composed of vascular loose connective tissue. The muscularis mucosa is composed of only a single layer of longitudinally oriented smooth muscle fibers. The submucosa is composed of loose connective tissue containing many blood vessels and esophageal glands (asterisk, Figure 12-1). Under the high power, the esophageal glands represent groups of small mucus-secreting gland whose secretion facilitates the transport of foodstuffs and protects the mucosa. The muscularis externa is made up of both skeletal and smooth muscle fibers. The upper one-third of the esophagus has mostly skeletal muscle; the

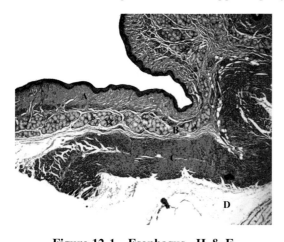

Figure 12-1　Esophagus, H & E
A: Mucosa; B: Submucosa; C: Muscularis externa;
D: Adventitia; Asterisk: Esophageal glands

middle one-third has both skeletal and smooth muscle; while the lowest one-third shows exclusively smooth muscle. What muscle type can you identify in the muscularis externa? The esophagus is covered externally by an adventitia. Question: What is the difference between serosa and adventitia?

2. Stomach (fundus or body), H & E

The fundus and body are identical in histological structure. They are the center of action in the stomach. At a low magnification, identify the four major layers of the wall i. e. mucosa, submucosa, muscularis externa and serosa (Figure 12-2). The mucosa is composed of the usual three components (Figure 12-3): epithelium, lamina propria and muscularis mucosa. Note that the mucosa is beset by many gastric pits.

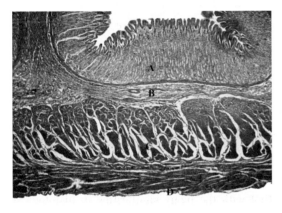

Figure 12-2　Stomach, H & E
A:Mucosa; B: Submucosa; C: Muscularis externa; D: Serosa

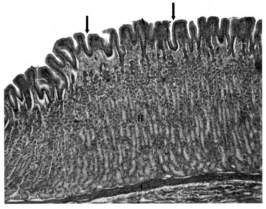

Figure 12-3　Stomach mucosa, H & E
A:Epithelium; B: Lamina propria; C: Muscularis mucosa; Black arrows: Gastric pits

Under the high power, the lining of the mucosa is simple columnar epithelium formed by the surface mucous epithelial cells. Note the absence of goblet cells in the gastric mucosa. The apical region of the surface mucous cells is palely stained cytoplasm and in some cells it appears as empty spaces (Figure 12-4). The lamina propria contains many fundic glands which open into the gastric pits. There are five types of cells in the fundic glands, and among them the parietal cells and chief cells are most numerous.

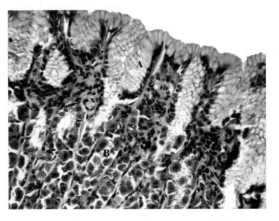

Figure 12-4　Stomach mucosa, H & E
A: Epithelium; B: Lamina propria

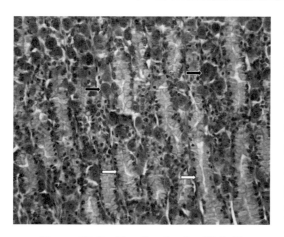

Figure 12-5　Fundic glands, H & E

Black arrows: Parietal cells; White arrows: Chief cells

The parietal cells (black arrow, Figure 12-5) are distributed mainly in the upper half of the gastric glands. They are large, pyramidal or spherical in shape. They are eosinophilic cells with a conspicuous centrally located nucleus. The cells resemble "fried eggs. " Parietal cells produce hydrochloric acid (HCl) and gastric intrinsic factor. Chief cells (white arrow, Figure 12-5) predominate in the lower half of the gastric glands. They are columnar, basophilic cells and are smaller than the parietal cells; they produce pepsinogen. Mucous neck cells are difficult to distinguish from the surface mucous epithelial cells.

3. Small intestine

The small intestine is the longest segment of the digestive tract and is divided into three segments: duodenum, jejunum and ileum. It is structured to provide a large surface area for absorption. Histological changes occur gradually in the transition from one segment to another. Before attempting to highlight the major differences between the three segments of the small intestine, you should familiarize yourself first with the many similarities in histological features shared by the different segments.

(1) Duodenum, H & E

First, orientate and examine the section with the naked eye. From the luminal side, note that the lining of the small intestine shows a series of folds, forming the plicae circularis (circular folds). Survey the entire section at a low magnification and then identify the four layers of the intestinal wall (Figure 12-6). Examine the prominent circular folds which are projections from the mucosa and submucosa. Are they as prominent as those found in the jejunum? The lamina propria is composed of loose connective tissue rich in lymphatic tissue, and numerous tubular small intestinal glands or crypts of Lierberkühn. Identify next the intestinal villi-projections of the epithelium and lamina propria in the mucosa. The submucosa is composed of connective tissue housing the duodenal glands also known as the Brunner's glands (Figure 12-6, Figure 12-7). The muscularis externa of the small intestine is composed of an inner circular layer and an outer longitudinal smooth muscle layer. The exterior of the duodenum is invested by a serosa with the exception for its second and third parts.

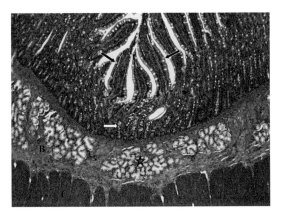

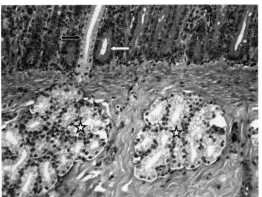

Figure 12-6   Duodenum, H & E

A: Mucosa; B: Submucosa; C: Muscularis externa;
Black arrows: Intestinal villi; White arrow: Intestinal gland (Crypts of Lierberkühn); Asterisk: Brunner's glands

Figure 12-7   Duodenum, H & E

Black arrow: Duct; White arrow: Intestinal gland;
Asterisk: Brunner's glands

Under the high power lens(Figure 12-8), the intestinal villi are tiny, finger-like projections that project from the epithelial lining of the intestinal wall into the lumen. The entire luminal surface is covered by the mucosa bearing large numbers of villi whose core is the lamina
propria that provides for a bedding support, and contents of blood vessels, nerves and lacteals. The epithelium (A, Figure 12-8) of the intestinal villus is simple columnar epithelium,
comprising the absorptive cells with a distinct layer of striated border (well-developed microvilli) facing the lumen (What is the functional significance of the striated border?), and
mucus-secreting goblet cells (black arrow, Figure 12-8). In what way is this different from
the epithelium of the stomach? The core of the villus is the lamina propria (B, Figure 12-8)
containing many connective tissue cells, blood capillaries, lacteals and lymphocytes.
Intestinal glands or crypts of Lierberkühn (Figure 12-7) are formed by invaginations of the
mucosa which extend beneath to reach almost the muscularis mucosa. They open between the
bases of the intestinal villi. Brunner's glands (or duodenal glands) are compound tubular
glands confined mainly to the submucosa of the duodenum (Figure 12-6, Figure 12-7). They
secrete alkaline mucus to neutralize the acid medium from the stomach.

(2) Jejunum, H & E

Identify the four main layers of its wall. In contrast to the duodenum, the jejunum has
very long finger-like villi and well-developed plica circularis (circular folds) which are projections from the mucosa and submucosa (Figure 12-9). The epithelium has a prominent striated border with more goblet cells. Note absence of Brunner's glands and Peyer's patches in
the submucosa.

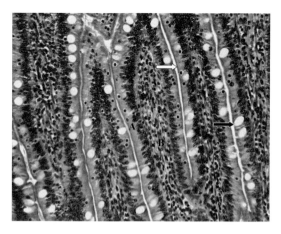

Figure 12-8　Duodenum, H & E

A：Epithelium；B：Lamina propria；White arrow：
Striated border；Black arrow：Goblet cell

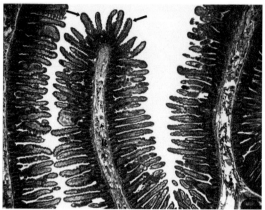

Figure 12-9　Jejunum, H & E

A：Mucosa；B：Submucosa；Black arrows：
Intestinal villi

（3）Ileum, H & E

The villi of the ileum are the least in numbers and shortest in comparison to other segments of the small intestine. The lamina propria houses a collection of lymphatic nodules, known as Peyer's patches. Peyer's patches may extend into the submucosa. Goblet cells are more numerous than the jejunum（Figure 12-10）.

4. Colon, H & E

Circular folds（plica circularis）or villi are absent in the colon；hence, the mucosal surface is relatively smooth. The surface is pitted with crypts of Lierberkühn（black arrow）, which contain a large number of goblet cells. The outer longitudinal layer of the muscularis externa varies in thickness. It is thickened regionally as three distinct longitudinal bands of muscle on the outer surface named as the "taenia coli" in gross anatomy（Figure 12-11）.

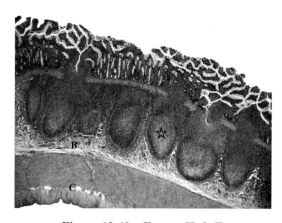

Figure 12-10　Ileum, H & E

A：Mucosa；B：Submucosa；C：Muscularis externa；
Asterisk：Peyer's patches

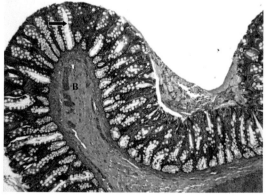

Figure 12-11　Colon, H & E

A：Mucosa；B：Submucosa；Black arrow：Crypts
of Lierberkühn

【Demonstration slides】

1. Tongue, H & E

The tongue is a muscular organ consisting of a core of interlacing skeletal muscle bundles. It is covered on its surface by a mucous membrane. (Question: What is the innervation to the tongue muscle?). The dorsal surface of the tongue in the anterior part is covered by a large number of small eminences called the lingual papillae. Filiform papillae are numerous and are present over the entire surface of the tongue (Figure 12-12). Fungiform papillae are randomly distributed among the filiform papillae. The surface epithelium is relatively thin and keratinized. Fungiform papillae contain scattered taste buds on their upper surfaces. Taste buds are barrel-shaped taste receptors extending the full thickness of the epithelium and opening at the surface via the taste pore.

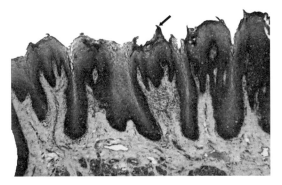

Figure 12-12   Tongue, H & E

Black arrow: Filiform papillae

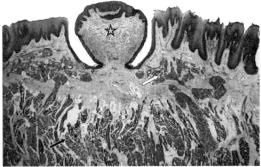

Figure 12-13   Tongue, H & E

Asterisk: A circumvallate papilla; White arrow: Serous von Ebner's glands; Black arrow: Tongue muscles (skeletal)

At the junction between the anterior and posterior one-third of the tongue and located immediately anterior to the sulcus terminalis are present 10 ~ 12 in number of cirucumvallate papillae. The cirumcumvallate papilla (Figure 12-13) is mushroom- shaped which is surrounded by a groove or trench and into which open the ducts of the serous von Ebner's glands (white arrow). The taste buds are located at the side of the papilla (Figure 12-14). Each taste bud contains sensory and supporting (sustentacular) cells. The taste buds associated with the circumvallate papilla are supplied by the glossopharyngeal nerve (IX cranial nerve).

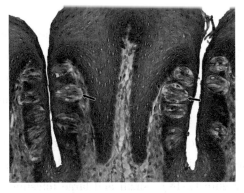

Figure 12-14   Tongue, H & E

Black arrows: Taste buds

2. Gastro-esophageal junction, H & E

The lining of the esophagus is stratified squamous epithelium but it changes abruptly into the simple columnar epithelium at the gastro-esophageal junction (Figure 12-15). In the stomach, the epithelium is entirely simple columnar which is beset by many gastric glands.

3. Pyloro-duodenal junction, H & E

In the pylorus on the left, globlet cells are absent. Identify the pylorus and note that the pyloric sphincter which is characterized by the presence of a thick layer of smooth muscle. What is the innervation of the pyloric sphincter muscle? The duodenum is on the right of the figure and is identified by the presence of Brunner's gland in the submucosa (Figure 12-16).

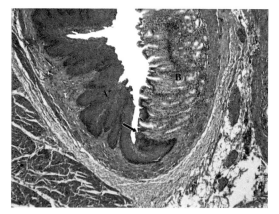

**Figure 12-15   Gastro-esophageal junction,
H & E**

A: Esophagus; B: Stomach; Black arrow: Gastro-esophageal junction

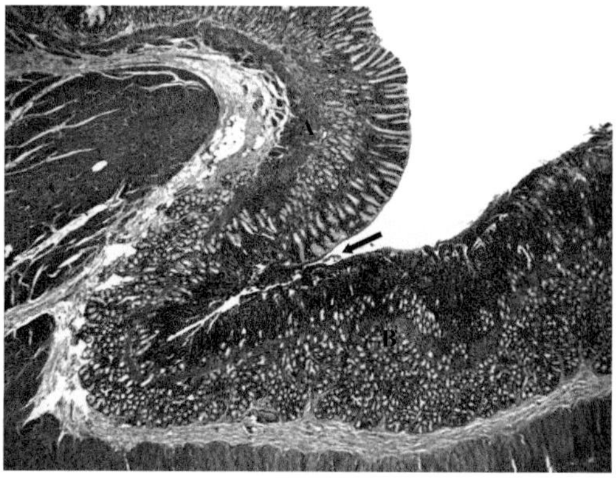

**Figure 12-16   Pyloro-duodenal junction,
H & E**

A: Pylorus; B: Duodenum; Black arrow: Pyloro-duodenal junction

4. Pyloric glands, H & E

Pyloric glands are located in the lamina propria in the pyloric region of the stomach. Just like the gastric glands in the body and fundus regions, the pyloric glands also open into the base of gastric pits. The epithelial cells are predominantly mucous cells, with a few scattered enteroendocrine cells and chief cells (Figure 12-17).

5. Endocrine cells, Stomach mucosa, Silver stain

The endocrine cells of the digestive system belong to the APUD (amine precursor uptake and decarboxylation) system. These cells are scattered in the epithelium of the stomach (Figure 12-18), small and large intestine.

6. Paneth cells, Small intestine, H & E

The cells are located at the base of the intestinal gland. They are laden with large, aci-dophilic, apical secretory granules containing lysozyme and zinc (Figure 12-19).

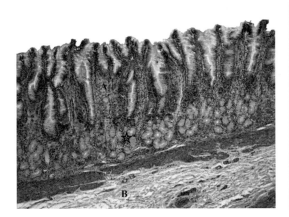

Figure 12-17   Pyloric glands, H & E

A: Mucosa; B: Submucosa; Asterisk: Pyloric
glands

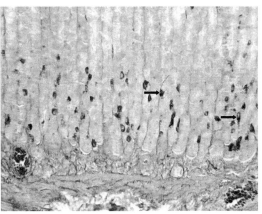

**Figure 12-18   Endocrine cells, Stomach
mucosa, Silver stain**

Black arrows: Endocrine cells

7. Appendix, H & E

The most distinctive feature of the appendix is the infiltration of massive lymphocytes into the lamina propria. The lymphatic nodules form almost a complete lymphoid ring that invades the submucosa. The muscularis externa and serosa have typical histological features shared by other parts of the digestive tract (Figure 12-20).

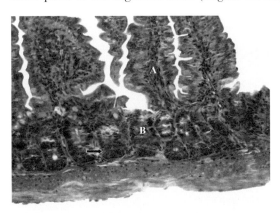

**Figure 12-19   Paneth cells, Small intestine,
H & E**

A: Intestinal villus; B: Intestinal gland; Black
arrow: Paneth cells

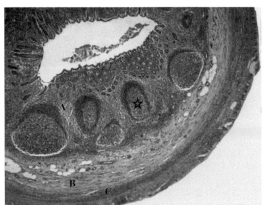

Figure 12-20   Appendix, H & E

A: Mucosa; B: Submucosa; C: Muscularis externa;
Asterisk: Lymphatic nodule

【Questions and clinical points for discussion and integration】

1. Describe the general histological structure of the digestive tract.

2. Describe the histology of the fundus of the stomach. What is the innervation of its muscles (muscularis externa and muscularis mucosa)?

3. Describe the structure and function of the small intestine. Highlight the histological

differences between the three parts of the small intestine.

4. Why is the mucosa of the stomach not eroded by hydrochloric acid and pepsin? What are the causes of gastric or peptic ulcer?

5. Highlight the histological differences between the small and large intestines.

6. Describe the histology of the appendix.

7. Describe the histology of the tongue, adding a note on its embryological development.

8. What is gastroscopy? What information may be gained from this procedure?

9. In acute appendicitis, where is the referred pain initially felt?

10. Based on your knowledge in gross anatomy and neuroanatomy, what is the basis of referred pain to the umbilical region (T10) in appendicitis?

(吴春云)

Chapter 13　Digestive Glands

The digestive glands associated with the digestive tract include three pairs of large salivary glands, pancreas and liver. The major salivary glands are the parotid, submandibular and sublingual glands which are derived from the primordial oral cavity during embryological development. Histologically, they are classified as the compound tubuloalveolar glands. The primary function of the digestive glands is to secrete digestive juice (liquid) containing a variety of digestive enzymes.

【Objectives】

1. To identify and describe:

A. submandibular gland (serous, mucous or seromucous acinus and ducts).

B. pancreas (exocrine pancreas, endocrine pancreas).

C. liver: anatomical lobule (hepatic lobule), central vein, hepatocyte plates, hepatocytes, hepatic sinusoids, macrophages (Kupffer cells), portal areas (portal triad), functional lobule (portal lobule).

2. To understand and describe the main histological features of the parotid and sublingual glands.

3. To understand and describe the histological structure of the gall bladder.

【Observation of tissue sections】

1. Submandibular gland, H & E

Survey the section of the submandibular gland under the low power and note the fibrous capsule at the surface. Nerves and blood vessels may be present in the capsule. Extending from the capsule into the parenchyma of the gland are a variable number of septa dividing the gland into many lobules. The basic secretory units of the submandibular gland are the serous acini, although there are present also some mucous acini. Between the secretory units is the branching duct system. Examine a lobule and locate first the intralobular ducts (striated and intercalated ducts within a lobule). The striated ducts appear in different planes of section: longitudinal, transverse or oblique. In view of the small lumen, the intercalated ducts are more difficult to identify.

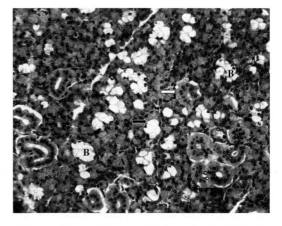

Figure 13-1　Submandibular gland, H & E
A:Serous alveoli; B: Mucous alveoli; Black arrow: Mixed alveoli; White arrow: Striated duct

The interlobular ducts are located in the connective tissue septa between the lobules. The interlobular duct is often accompanied by blood vessels. Examine the acini under the high power objective lens. There are three types of acini: serous, mucous and mixed acinus (Figure 13-1).

(1) Serous acinus: It is composed of serous cells, usually pyramidal in shape, whose broad cell base rests on a layer of basal lamina. The apical cell surface is narrow facing a small lumen in the center of the acinus. The serous cells have a round basal nucleus. In the basal region, the granular cytoplasm tends to be basophilic but it appears more eosinophilic than in the apical area. Serous cells are protein-secreting cells.

(2) Mucous acinus: It is formed by the mucous cells which are usually cuboidal to columnar in shape. The nucleus is either flattened or oval and is often located near to the base of the cells. Mucous cells are mucus-secreting cells, containing large numbers of mucinogen granules in the apical cytoplasm. The mucinogen is lost in H&E stained sections; hence, the apical portion of the cell usually appears empty looking. Note the characteristic features of the serous and mucous acini. How do you differentiate the two types of acini?

(3) Mixed acinus: It contains both serous and mucous cells. In H&E staining sections, the mucous acinus is capped by a small cluster of serous cells in crescent shaped called the serous demilune.

2. Pancreas, H & E

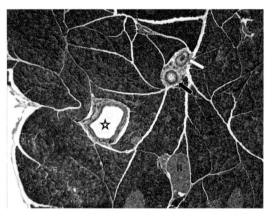

Figure 13-2　Pancreas, H & E
A:Pancreatic acini, B: Pancreatic islets; Black arrow:
Artery; White arrow: Vein; Asterisk: Interlobular duct

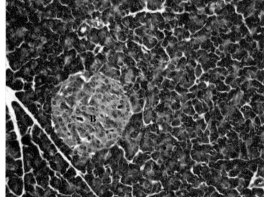

Figure 13-3　Pancreas, H & E
A:Pancreatic acini; B: Pancreatic islet (Islet of
Langerhans)

The pancreas is covered by a thin layer of connective tissue which sends septa into the parenchyma, subdividing it into numerous small lobules (Figure 13-2). The interlobular connective tissue is scanty. Intralobular ducts are evident. Identify the lobular pattern which is similar to a serous salivary gland. Pancreas has both exocrine and endocrine in function. The exocrine portion is represented by abundant, tubulo-alveolar serous acini. Observe the sectional profiles of ducts of various sizes. The pancreatic acini are round or slightly elongated, and are made up of pyramidal acinar cells around a small lumen. The acinar cells have a spherical nucleus, which lies near the base of the cell, and an intensely stained basophilic cytoplasm. The cytoplasm in the apical region of the acinar cells is filled with closely packed secretory granules called the zymogen granules. Identify the centro-acinar cells under high power. What do they secrete?

The endocrine pancreas is represented by islets of Langerhans (Figure 13-2, Figure 13-3). Often, the islets are difficult to identify, but characteristically they are seen at lower power as lightly stained, rounded masses of anastomosing cords of specialized epithelial cells, separated by capillaries. Individual islet cells (i. e. α, β, δ, PP cells) are not distinguishable in H&E preparation.

3. Liver (pig), H & E

The anatomical hepatic lobules are readily identifiable in the pig's liver (Figure 13-4). This is because the organ contains a lot of connective tissue which delineates the individual lobules. First, note that the surface of the liver is covered by a distinct layer of connective tissue. Next, familiarize yourself with the characteristic histologic features of the liver such as the portal triad comprising the small branches of the portal vein, hepatic artery, and bile ductule. Some lymphatic vessels may also be seen in the triad area. They are smaller in diameter than the blood vessels but are devoid of red blood cells. Locate the central vein, hepatic plates (hepatocytes), and sinusoids (Figure 13-5).

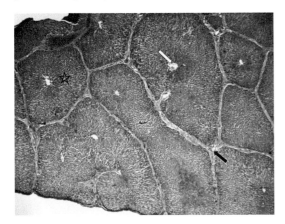

Figure 13-4   Liver (pig), H & E
Asterisk: Hepatic lobule; Black arrow: Portal
area; White arrow: Central vein

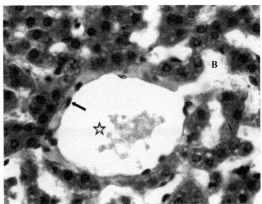

**Figure 13-5   Hepatic lobule, Liver (pig),
H & E**
Asterisk: Central vein; Black arrow: Endothe-
lium; A: Hepatic cord; B: Sinusoid

(1) Central vein: This may be considered the terminal hepatic venule with numerous pores in its very thin walls. It receives blood from the sinusoids with blood derived from the hepatic artery as well as the portal vein.

(2) Hepatic plates: These anastomosing hepatic plates are made up of rows of hepatic cells (hepatocytes). Between the hepatic plates are tiny anastomosing secretory channels called the bile canaliculi. In a histologic section (transverse section), the hepatic plates ap-

pear as interconnecting cords of cells of one or two-cell thick, called hepatocyte cords separated by hepatic sinusoids. The hepatic plates radiate from the central vein toward the periphery of the lobule. Under the high power, hepatocytes are large polygonal cells with one or two large and round nuclei and prominent nucleoli; the acidophilic cytoplasm may contain some basophilic granules.

(3) Hepatic sinusoids: These are large and irregular radiations extending from the central vein in a lobule and forming an extensive spongy network. Liver macrophages, called Kupffer cells are situated in the sinusoids. Endothelial cells and Kupffer cells are associated with the sinusoidal lining. The hepatic plates are separated by sinusoids which appear empty looking. They were filled with blood but had been washed away during slide preparation. Identify the perisinusoidal space (space of Disse) present between the sinusoidal endothelium and adjacent hepatocytes.

(4) Portal areas (triad): These are found at the angles between adjacent hepatic lobules, containing connective tissue and several ducts (Figure 13-6).

● Interlobular artery: it is a branch of hepatic artery, and has the features typical of that of a small muscular artery.

● Interlobular vein: it is a tributary of portal vein, and shows the histological features of a small vein.

● Interlobular bile duct: the lumen is lined by a simple cuboidal or low columnar epithelium.

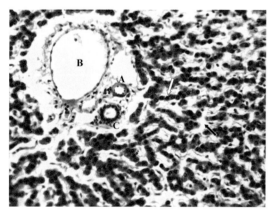

Figure 13-6 Portal area (triad), H & E
A: Interlobular artery; B: Interlobular vein; C: Interlobular bile duct; White arrow: Hepatic cord; Black arrow: Sinusoid

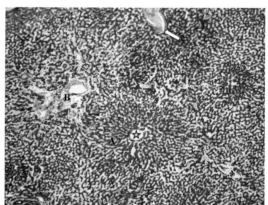

Figure 13-7 Liver (monkey), H & E
A: Hepatic lobule; B: Portal area (triad); Asterisk: Central vein; White arrow: Sublobularvein

4. Liver (monkey), H & E

Survey your section under the low power. Note the lack of distinct boundaries between different lobules, and that the lobules are not separated by a layer of connective tissue (Figure 13-7). Portal triad is an irregular-shaped area between adjacent hepatic lobules.

The architecture of the liver can be described in two ways. Try to understand the relationship between the anatomical and functional lobules. The anatomical lobule with the central vein in the center is useful for the study of liver morphology, but it does not give much information about the functional units of the liver. In a functional lobule in which the portal triad lies in the center, blood flows from the center in all directions toward the neighboring central veins. Such an arrangement or configuration would offer a better explanation for some liver diseases. For example, reduced arterial blood supply would manifest itself initially by affecting the cells nearest the central vein, while toxic substances in the blood would show up first in cells near the portal triad.

【Demonstration slides】

1. Parotid gland, H & E

The parotid gland is exclusively serous, with long intercalated ducts and short striated ducts. The covering capsule, septa, lobules and ducts are similar to the other mixed salivary glands (Figure 13-8). Questions: What is mumps? Review the secretomotor innervation of the major salivary glands. Which cranial nerve is closely associated with the parotid gland and which may be damaged in parotid surgery?

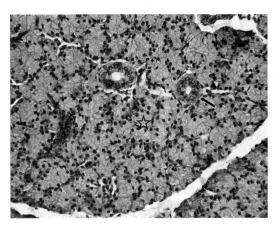

Figure 13-8　Parotid gland, H & E
Asterisk: Serous alveoli; Black arrow: Intralobular duct
(Striated duct)

2. Sublingual gland, H & E

The sublingual gland is made up almost entirely of mucous acini. Some mucous acini are occasionally capped by a serous demilune (a piece of crescent shaped serous acinar tissue) (Figure 13-9). Question: How is the secretion from the serous demilune released into the lumen of the acinus? Why is the striated duct so named?

3. Kupffer cells, Liver

Under the low power, identify the "red cells" which are the hepatic macrophages (Kupffer cells) in the sinusoids. The cells have ingested red foreign particles which were earlier introduced into the blood circulation (Figure 13-10).

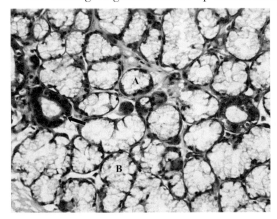

Figure 13-9　Sublingual gland, H & E
A: mixed alveoli; B: Mucous alveoli; Black arrow:
Intralobular duct (Striated duct)

4. Bile canaliculi, Silver stain

Using the high power objective lens, you should be able to identify small dark spots or thread-like structures between the hepatocytes, the bile canaliculi (Figure 13-11).

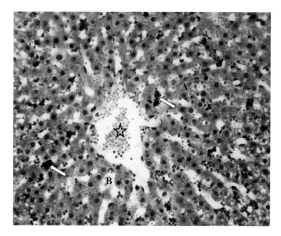

Figure 13-10　Kupffer cells, H & E

Asterisk: Central vein; A: Hepatic cords; B: Sinusoid; White arrows: Kupffer cells

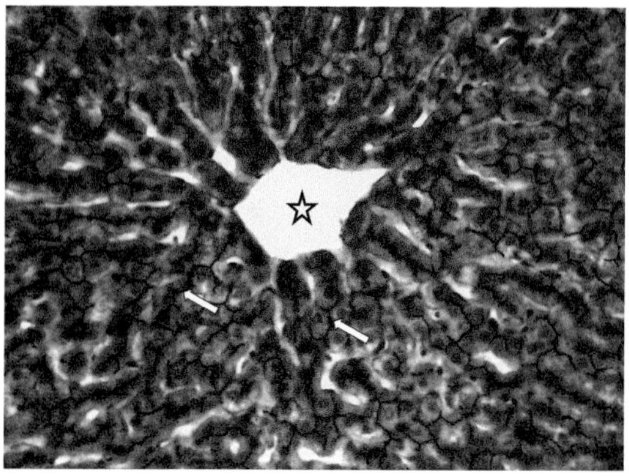

Figure 13-11　Bile canaliculi, Silver stain

Asterisk: Central vein; White arrows: Bile canaliculi

【Questions and clinical points for discussion and integration】

1. List the major histological differences between the salivary glands and the pancreas.

2. Describe the histological structure and function of pancreas (exocrine pancreas, endocrine pancreas).

3. What is acute hemorrhagic necrotizing pancreatitis (ANNP)?

4. Review the major functions of the liver.

5. Describe the histological structure of an anatomic hepatic lobule.

6. Based on your knowledge of cytology, which organelle would be well developed in hepatocytes?

7. Where do Kupffer cells originate? What organelle is prominent in these cells?

8. What is the definition of a portal system? Do you find any other portal system in the body?

9. Appreciate that blood from the hepatic artery mixes with that of the portal vein in the hepatic sinusoids and central vein.

10. What is obstructive jaundice?

11. Review the histology of the gall bladder. What is the main function of this organ?

(赵　敏)

Chapter 14　Respiratory System

The respiratory system consists of two main portions with distinctive functions: an air-conducting portion and a respiratory portion. The trachea and the paired lungs are the key structures of this system.

【Objectives】

1. To identify and describe:

A. trachea: mucosa, submucosa (seromucous glands), adventitia.

B. lung: the conducting portion (bronchus, bronchiole, terminal bronchiole) and the respiratory portion (respiratory bronchiole, alveolar duct, alveolar sac, and alveolus).

2. To relate the histological changes of the bronchial tree to its functions.

【Observation of tissue sections】

1. Trachea, H & E

The tracheal wall is composed of three tunics (layers): mucosa, submucosa and adventitia. Identify the various layers in the wall of the trachea.

Mucosa (A, Figure 14-1) consists of the epithelium and the laminar propria. The lining epithelium is pseudostratified ciliated columnar epithelium or simply, the respiratory epithelium. What are the constituent cells of the epithelium? Identify the ciliated cells

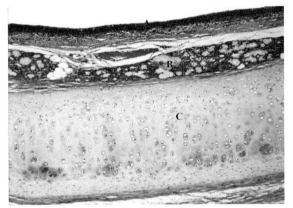

Figure 14-1　Trachea, H & E

A: Mucosa; B: Submucosa (with serous mucous glands);

C: Adventitia

(cilia on their free surface) and goblet cells (goblet in shape and filled with mucinogen droplets). What is the specific function of each of the cell types? Beneath the epithelium is the lamina propria, composed of connective tissue with abundant elastic fibers, smooth muscle bundles and lymphatic tissue. Seromucous glands (serous and mucous) and blood vessels are present in the submucosa (B, Figure 14-1). Identify the C-shaped hyaline cartilage ring supporting the wall in the adventitia (C, Figure 14-1). The posterior gap is bridged by a fibro-elastic membrane and smooth muscle (trachealis muscle). What is its function? Blood vessels, nerves, lymphatics and adipose tissue may be found in the adventitia.

2. Lung, H & E

The main (primary) bronchus, after entering the lungs, branches repeatedly to form the bronchial tree; the end branches finally terminate at the alveoli.

(1) Conducting portion: intrapulmonary bronchi (secondary/lobar bronchi, and

tertiary/segmental bronchi). Note a lobar bronchus supplies a specific lobe (upper, middle or lower) of the lung, while a segmental bronchus supplies a bronchopulmonary segment (normally 10 on the right lung, 8 on the left). The intrapulmonary bronchi may be hard to find in the slide allocated to you. Refer to your histology atlas for better illustration. The bronchus continues as the bronchioles (<1mm), and then terminal bronchioles (<0.5mm).

The conducting portion of the lung undergoes progressive morphologic changes when traced distally. The first change is the decrease in luminal diameter. Identify the epithelium lining the lumen. Note the prominent cilia on the columnar cells. Question: What forms the core of a cilium? Can you recognize the cartilage plates? What type of cartilage is found in the bronchus cartilage plates? Do you find a layer of perichondrium? Locate next the sero-mucous glands.

The following are some highlights of the major histological changes with the branching of the conducting portion of the lung:

a. Epithelium: Pseudostratified ciliated columnar (thick → thin) → simple ciliated columnar →simple columnar.

b. Goblet cells: more → few → absent.

c. Glands: more → few → absent.

d. Cartilage plates: more, large → few, small → absent.

e. Smooth muscle: scattered bundles → relatively more, thick → circular layer.

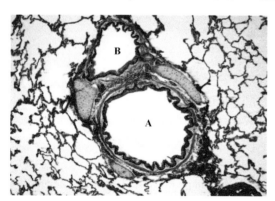

Figure 14-2   Lung, H & E
A: Bronchus; B: Bronchiole

1) Bronchus:As in trachea, the epithelium is pseudostratified ciliated columnar epithelium, but the C-shaped cartilage is replaced by discontinuous plates of cartilage. Smooth muscle and occasional glandular tissue may be seen. The bronchi differ in size and amount of cartilage (A, Figure 14-2).

2) Bronchiole: It has a smaller diameter than the bronchus but it lacks cartilage or glands. The lining epithelium is simple ciliated or non-ciliated columnar. Contraction of the smooth muscle causes the bronchiolar wall to have a "ruffled" appearance in cross-section, called circular mucosa folds or plical folds (B, Figure 14-2; A, Figure 14-3). Question: What is the innervation to the bronchiolar smooth muscle? Which neurotransmitter causes its contraction? What is asthma? What is the nerve supply to the mucous membrane of the bronchi and bronchioles?

3) Terminal bronchiole: It is considered the distal part of a bronchiole before it opens into the respiratory bronchiole which is partly lined by alveoli. The epithelium is simple columnar or

simple cuboidal epithelium. The goblet cells, sero-mucous glands and cartilage plates are diminished or absent. The smooth muscles form a complete circular layer (B, Figure 14-3).

(2) Respiratory portion: Respiratory bronchioles, alveolar ducts, alveolar sacs, and alveoli (Figure 14-3, Figure 14-4). These segments are involved in exchange of gases.

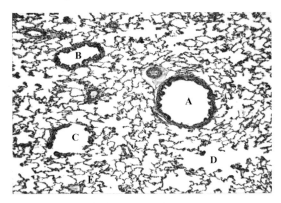

Figure 14-3   Lung, H & E
A: Bronchiole; B: Terminal bronchiole; C: Respiratory bronchiole; D: Alveolar duct; E: Alveolar sac

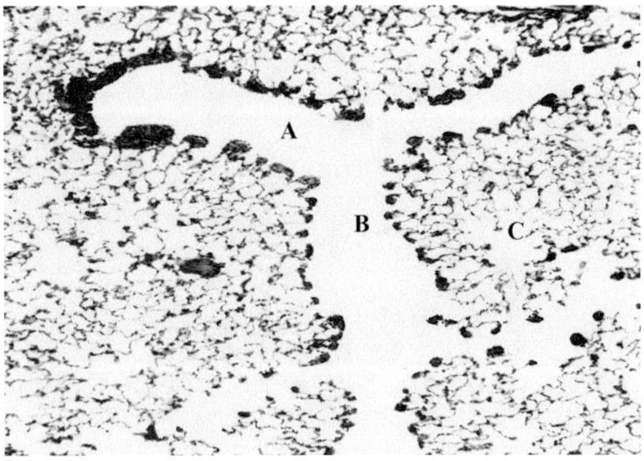

Figure 14-4   Lung, H & E
A: Respiratory bronchiole; B: Alveolar duct; C: Alveolar sac

1) Respiratory bronchiole: The respiratory bronchiole is a transitional area involved in both gas conduction and gas exchange. The wall is interrupted by scattered, thin-walled outpocketings (alveoli), hence, is lined by simple squamous epithelium; elsewhere, it is lined by simple cuboidal epithelium.

2) Alveolar ducts: The alveolar duct is an elongated passage with many alveoli, which share a central, duct-like space. The wall between adjacent alveoli which appears as knobs is lined by simple squamous epithelium.

3) Alveolar sacs: These are clusters of alveoli that have a common opening of spherical central space.

4) Alveoli: They are the thin-walled polygonal compartments and the sites of gas exchange. The alveolus is lined by two types of alveolar epithelial cells (Type I and II pneumocytes) (black arrow and white arrow, Figure 14-5).

5) Interalveolar septum: This lies between two adjacent alveoli. It contains an extensive network of capillaries, elastic

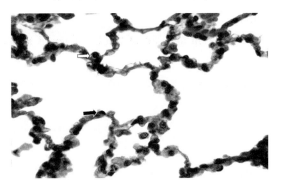

Figure 14-5   Alveoli, Lung, H & E
Black arrow: Type I pneumocyte; White arrow: Type II pneumocye

fibers and clusters of alveolar macrophages (present in the inter-alveolar septum or alveolar lumen, also called the "dust cells" with internalized dust particles) (black arrow, Figure 14-6).

【Demonstration slide】

Tracheal epithelial cells, H & E

They are ciliated columnar cells. Cilia can be seen (black arrows, Figure 14-7).

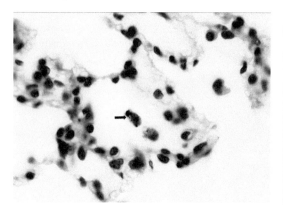

Figure 14-6   Alveoli, Lung, H & E

Black arrow: Dust cell

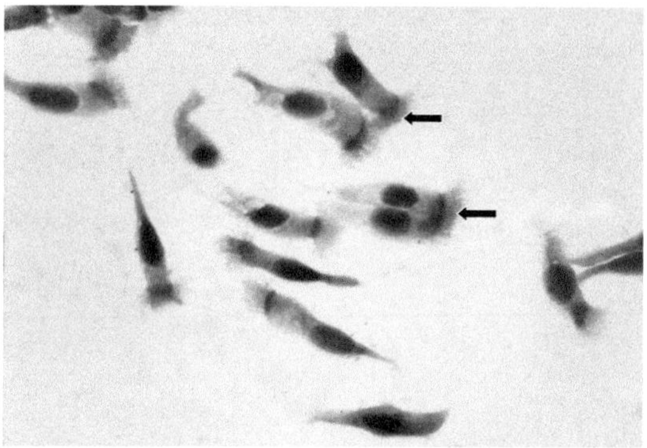

Figure 14-7   Trachea epithelial cells, H & E

Black arrow: Ciliated columnar cells

【Questions and clinical points for discussion and integration】

1. Discuss the histological basis of chronic obstructive pulmonary disease (COPD).

2. Discuss the innervation of the lung.

3. What is the histological/neuroanatomical/pharmacological basis for asthma?

4. What is bronchiectasis?

5. Compare the differences in histology and functions between the bronchus and bronchiole.

6. Describe the structure of an inter-alveolar septum and relate this to its respiratory function.

7. Give an account of the histology of the trachea.

(马丽梅)

Chapter 15　Urinary System

The urinary system consists of the paired kidneys and ureters, the unpaired bladder and urethra. Urine produced in the kidneys passes through the ureters to the bladder, where it is temporarily stored and then released to the exterior through the urethra. In this histological practical class, the histological structure of the kidney is emphasized. The nephron is the functional unit of the kidney.

【Objectives】

1. To identify and describe:

A. the renal corpuscle, proximal convoluted tubule, thin part of loop of Henle, and distal convoluted tubule, macula densa.

B. the histological structure of the collecting duct.

2. To briefly describe the structure of the proximal straight tubule and distal straight tubule.

3. To understand and describe the histological structure of the ureter and the bladder and relate this to their functions.

【Observation of tissue section】

Kidney, H & E

Examine the section with the naked eye. The approximate boundary between the cortex (dark) and the medulla (pale) can be demarcated.

Under the low magnification (Figure 15-1), the kidney surface is covered by a connective tissue capsule. The substance of the kidney can be divided into two distinct regions: an outer cortex and an inner medulla.

A low power light micrograph shows a small area of the renal cortex (Figure 15-2). The cortex is organized into a series of medullary rays containing closely packed straight tubules and collecting tubules, and between them the cortical labyrinths containing the renal corpuscles and their associated tubules.

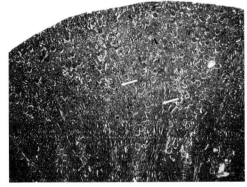

Figure 15-1　Kidney, H & E

A:Cortex; B: Medulla; White arrows: Medullary rays

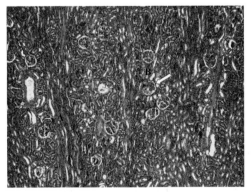

Figure 15-2　Renal cortex, Kidney, H & E

A:Medullary rays; B: Cortical labyrinths; White arrow: Renal corpuscle

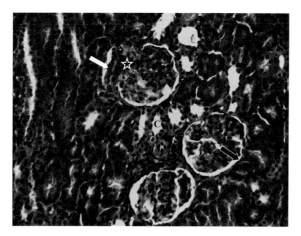

Figure 15-3　Renal cortex, Kidney, H & E

A：Renal glomerulus；B：Proximal convoluted tubule (PCT)；
C：Distal convoluted tubule (DCT)；White arrow：Macula
densa；Black arrow：Bowman's capsule；Asterisk：extraglomer-
ular mesangial cells

A high power light micrograph of the renal cortex is shown in Figure 15-3. The cortex is characterized by the presence of renal corpuscles, and their associated proximal and distal convoluted tubules. Each renal corpuscle is composed of the renal glomerulus (A, Figure 15-3) and glomerular (Bowman's) capsule (black arrow, Figure 15-3), which is surrounded by a double-walled epithelial capsule. The internal layer (the visceral layer and its modified lining cells called podocytes) envelops the capillaries of the glomerulus. The external layer forms the outer limit of the renal corpuscle and is called the parietal layer of Bowman's capsule. Note the flattened cells of the parietal layer. Can you recognize the epithelium? Between the two layers of Bowman's capsule is the Bowman's space.

Between the renal corpuscles are various profiles of proximal convoluted tubules (PCT) and distal convoluted tubules (DCT). The PCT is longer than the DCT, hence, the sectional profiles are more frequently seen near the renal corpuscles in the renal cortex. The cells of the cuboidal epithelium show an acidophilic cytoplasm. The cell apex has a "brush border" (Recall what this is under the electron microscope). The DCT is lined by a layer of simple cuboidal epithelium whose lining cells are flatter and smaller than those of the PCT. It is paler in staining and has indistinct brush border. The macula densa may be identified (white arrow,

Figure 15-3) at the vascular pole of a renal corpuscle. It contains modified cells of the distal tubule at the juxtaglomerular region. The cells usually assume a columnar form characterized by their closely packed nuclei. They serve as chemoreceptors sensing the changes of Na^+ ions that pass along. Identify the extraglomerular mesangial cells (lacis cells) wedged between the macula densa and the vascular pole of the renal corpuscle (asterisk, Figure 15-3). The function of lacis cells is unclear. The

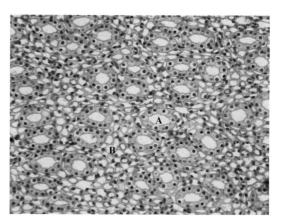

Figure 15-4　Renal medulla, Kidney, H & E

A：Collecting tubule；B：Thin segment of loop of Henle

cells are thought to play a part in transmission of signal from the macula densa to the intraglomerular mesangial cells.

Move your field now to the corticomedullary junction. Locate the arcuate arteries (cut transversely). At a high magnification of the medulla (Figure 15-4), identify the collecting tubules/ducts, and the thin segment of loop of Henle. The smaller collecting tubules are lined by cuboidal epithelium and their cells increase in height until they become columnar. Along their entire extent, the collecting tubules and ducts are composed of cells that are weakly stained. Note the distinct cell boundaries between the lining cells of the collecting tubules and ducts. The wall of the thin segment of loop of Henle consists of simple squamous epithelial cells whose nuclei bulges slightly into the lumen. The thick descending limb (proximal straight tubule) and thick ascending limb (distal straight tubule) loops of Henle display histological features similar to the proximal convoluted tubule and distal convoluted tubule, respectively, except that they are arranged in parallel arrays along with the collecting tubules. The straight tubules are located near the corticomedullary junction.

【Demonstration slides】

1. Blood vessels in the renal cortex

Photomicrograph showing the blood vessels (dark) in the renal cortex (Figure 15-5). The interlobular arteries give off branches forming the afferent arterioles. The afferent arterioles give rise to the capillaries that form the glomerulus. The dark reticular structures around the glomerulus are the second capillary network (peritubular).

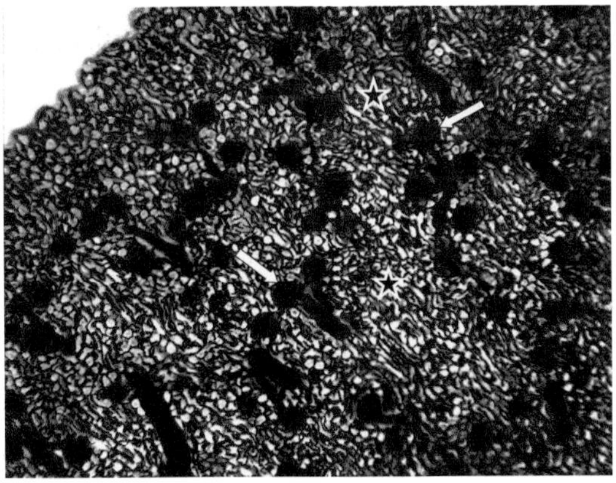

Figure 15-5 Blood vessels in the renal cortex

White arrows: Glomeruli; Asterisks: Second capillary networks

2. Ureter, H & E

A low power photomicrographof the ureter in transverse section (Figure 15-6). The wall of the ureter is composed of three layers: mucosa, muscularis layer and adventitia. The muscular layer consists of an inner longitudinal and an outer circular smooth muscle layer.

A low power photomicrograph of the urinary bladder wall (Figure 15-7). The urinary bladder is structurally similar to the ureter except for the smooth muscle layer which is much thicker. Identify the mucosa showing a transitional epithelium lining. The thick muscular layer (detrusor muscle) consists of interlacing smooth muscle fibers.

A high magnification image of the urinary bladder (Figure 2-10, Figure 2-11). Transitional epithelium (urothelium) lines the luminal surface of the wall of the bladder. The top layered cells are also called the "facet cells" whose plasma membrane facing the lumen forms a protective barrier against the hyperosmotic urine.

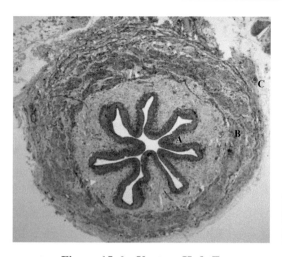

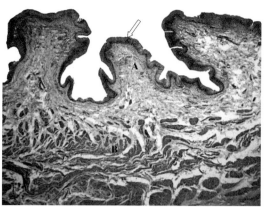

Figure 15-6   Ureter, H & E

A: Mucosa; B: Muscularis layer; C: Adventitia

Figure 15-7   Urinary bladder, H & E

A: Mucosa; B: Muscularis layer; White arrow: Transitional epithelium

【Questions and clinical points for discussion and integration】

1. Describe the structure of a nephron and relate its different parts to their specific functions.

2. Describe the histological differences between the ureter and the vas deferens.

3. Give an account of the juxtaglomerular complex mentioning its structural and functional components. What are the functions of the various components?

4. Describe the histology of the bladder. What is its parasympathetic nerve supply?

5. Name the three parts of the male urethra. What is the lining epithelium of each part?

6. Where do the renal arteries originate? How does the left renal artery differ from the right one?

7. What functional disorder may result if the renal artery is narrowed?

8. Give an account of the rennin angiotensin system.

9. If a stone is lodged in the ureter, peristaltic contraction of the muscle will cause excruciating pain (ureteric colic). Where is the pain referred to on the body surface i. e. area of dermatome that the pain may be felt? How do you relieve the ureteric colic pain? Where are the sites that the stone in the ureter are likely to be impacted?

10. What is the nerve supply to the muscle (detrusor) of urinary bladder?

11. What are the unique or specialized features of the top layer cells (facet cells) of the transitional epithelium?

12. Why is female more prone to urinary tract infection?

(曾园山)

Chapter 16　Endocrine System

The endocrine system comprises glands and tissues composed of parenchymal cells, which synthesize and secrete products called hormones that act on target tissues or cells far removed from the source of their production. The endocrine system has diverse regulatory functions that control and coordinate activities of many other organs and tissues. The major endocrine glands include the pituitary (or hypophysis ; considered as the "Leader of Endocrine Orchestra") , thyroid, parathyroid, adrenal and pineal gland. Most endocrine glands consist of a covering capsule and parenchymal cells. They are rich in vascular supply composed of a network of fenestrated capillaries.

【Objectives】

1. To identify and describe:

A. thyroid gland: follicular- and parafollicular (calcitonin) cells.

B. adrenal gland: cortex and medulla, zona fasciculata, zona glomerulosa and zona reticularis.

C. pituitary gland: pars distalis (chromophils and chromophobes), pars intermedia, and pars nervosa.

2. To understand and describe the main histological structure of the parathyroid gland, and its hormone and actions.

3. To understand and describe the histological structure of the endocrine part of the pancreas (Islets of Langerhans) , and its hormones and actions.

【Observation of tissue sections】

1. Thyroid & Parathyroid gland, H & E

The capsule coversthe parenchyma of the gland (Figure 16-1). Identify the thyroid follicles of various sizes filled with colloid and the interfollicular connective tissue. Spherical follicles are lined by simple cuboidal epithelium, which consists of vast majority of thyroid follicular cells and a few parafollicular (calcitonin) cells (Figure 16-2). The parafollicular cells are larger and paler than the follicular cells, and they exist as single cell or small clusters, in the follicular epithelium or in the interstitium between the follicles. The lumen of the follicle is filled with gelatinous colloid made up of thyroglobulin that shows a homogeneous appearance.

A portion of the parathyroid gland may also be seen in the same section (Figure 16-3). The connective tissue capsule sends a variable number of trabeculae into the parenchyma. Identify the chief cells (principal cells) and also oxyphil cells (with acidophilic cytoplasm) in the parathyroid gland (Figure 16-4). The chief cells are arranged in irregular cords. Oxyphil cells occur infrequently and often exist singly or in small cell clusters. They are larger and may have distinct cell boundaries.

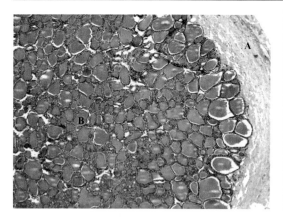

Figure 16-1 Thyroid , H & E

A: Capsule; B: Thyroid follicles

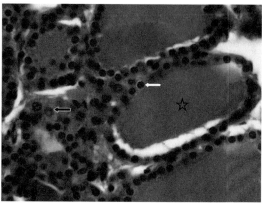

Figure 16-2 Thyroid , H & E

White arrow: follicular cell; Black arrow: Parafollicular cell; Asterisk: Follicle lumen

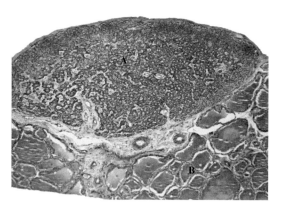

**Figure 16-3 Thyroid & Parathyroid gland ,
H & E**

A: Parathyroid gland; B: Thyroid gland

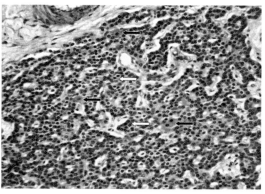

Figure 16-4 Parathyroid gland , H & E

White arrows: Chief cells; Black arrows: Oxyphil cells

2. Adrenal gland (Suprarenal gland) , H & E

Identify the fibrous connective tissue capsule and trabeculae, cortex and medulla (Figure
16-5).

Identify the three zones of the cortex from outside inwards (zona glomerulosa, zona fasciculata and zona reticularis) (Figure 16-6). The zona glomerulosa, lying immediately deep
to the capsule, is made up of closely packed, rounded clusters of parenchymal cells. The
middle zona fasciculata consisting of mainly radially oriented cords of polyhedral cells is in
close relation to fenestrated capillaries or sinusoids. These cells contain many lipid droplets,
which give the cytoplasm a pale foamy appearance. The thin innermost zona reticularis is composed of smaller, more acidophilic parenchymal cells arranged as an anastomosing network of
short cords with intervening sinusoidal capillaries. Review the hormones synthesized by the
cells of the adrenal cortex. The medulla is in the center of the gland, which contains cords or
nests of polyhedral chromaffin cells (stained by chromium salt, and hence its name) surroun-

ded by fenestrated capillaries. What are the secretions of the cells in the medulla? Sectional profiles of small venules are widely distributed in the medulla. A larger one which may represent the central vein of the medulla is indicated by an asterisk. Some red blood cells may be seen in the vessel. What is the embryological origin of the adrenal medulla?

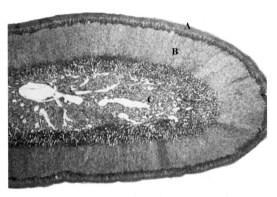

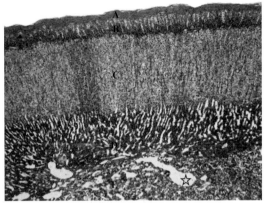

Figure 16-5   Adrenal gland, H & E

A: Capsule; B: Cortex; C: Medulla

Figure 16-6   Adrenal gland, H & E

A: Capsule; B: Zona glomerulosa; C: Zona fasciculata;
D: Zona reticularis; E: Medulla; Asterisk: Central vein

3. Pituitary gland, H & E

Examine the slide with the naked eye. The darker portion is the pars distalis, the paler portion is the pars nervosa, and the portion between them is the pars intermedia (Figure 16-7). Under Low power objective lens (Figure 16-8), locate the pars distalis, pars intermedia and pars nervosa.

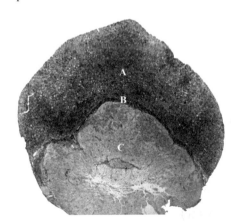

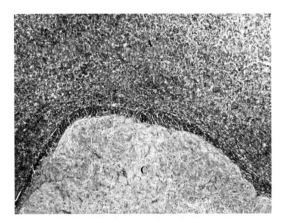

Figure 16-7   Pituitary gland, H & E

A: Pars distalis; B: Pars intermedia; C: Pars nervosa

Figure 16-8   Pituitary gland, H & E

A: Pars distalis; B: Pars intermedia; C: Pars nervosa

In the pars distalis (Figure 16-9), and under high power objective lens, identify the following cell types: chromophobes and chromophils; acidophils and basophils. What are the hormones synthesized by the chromophils (acidophils and basophils)? Numerous blood

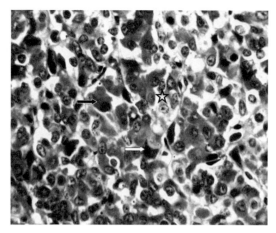

Figure 16-9   Pars distalis, Pituitary gland, H & E

White arrow: Basophil; Black arrow: Acidophil; Asterisk: Chromophobes

vessels (sinusoids) containing red blood cells are present.

Pars nervosa (asterisk, Figure 16-10) contains numerous nerve fibres (unmyelinated axons from the neurosecretory cells located in the hypothalamic nuclei paraventricular nucleus [PVN] and supraoptic nucleus [SON]) and pituicytes (These are modified astrocytes) (Figure 16-10). Appreciate that the pars nervosa is anatomically and functionally connected to the hypothalamic nuclei (supraoptic nucleus, SON and paraventricular nucleus, PVN) via "secretory axons" from the cell bodies of the hypothalamus. "Herring bodies" (eosinophilic colloid, black arrow) may be seen in the pars nervosa and they represent secretory material accumulated at intervals along each axon before being released into blood circulation. Question: What do "Herring bodies" contain?

【Demonstration slides】

1. **Parafollicular cells, Silver stain**

Under high power objective lens, the dark brown cells are parafollicular cells (white arrow, Figure 16-11) in the follicular epithelium or between the follicles (asterisk, Figure 16-11). What is their secretion?

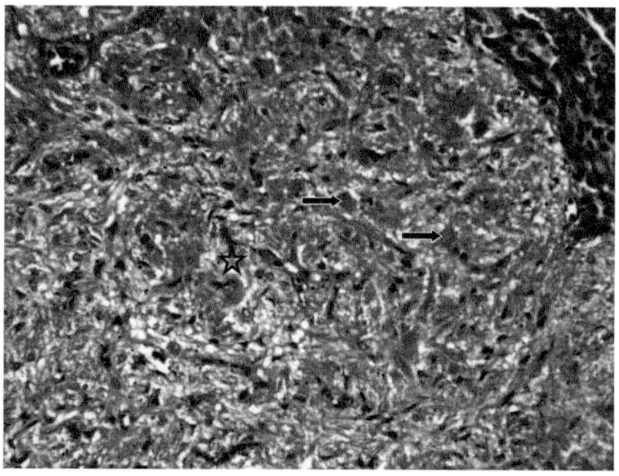

2. **Cells in the pars distalis, Special stain**

Under high power objective lens (Figure 16-12), identify the red cells

Figure 16-10   Pars nervosa, Pituitary gland, H & E

Asterisk: Pars nervosa; Black arrows: Herring bodies

which are acidophils; the blue cells, basophils, and the pale cells, chromophobes.

【Questions and topics for discussion and integration】

1. What are the common histological features of endocrine glands?

2. Describe the histology of the neurohypophysis. How is it connected to the hypothalamus structurally and functionally? Name the hormones secreted by it. What are the target cells or tissues of these hormones?

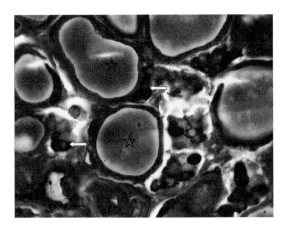

Figure 16-11   Parafollicular cells, Silver stain

White arrows: Parafollicular cells; Asterisks:
Thyroid follicles

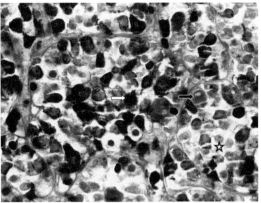

**Figure 16-12   Pars distalis, Pituitary gland,
Special stain**

Black arrow: Basophil; White arrow: Acidophil; Asterisk: Chromophobes

3. Name the parts of the adenohypophysis. What are the component cells and what are their secretions?

4. Describe the histology of the thyroid gland. How is thyroglobulin synthesized by the organ? Where is site of iodination of thyroglobulin?

5. Describe the histology of the adrenal (suprarenal) gland. What are its secretions and their actions?

6. Describe the endocrine part of the pancreas. What are the types of diabetes? Explain the histological basis for this.

(袁 云)

Chapter 17　Male Reproductive System

The male reproductive system comprises the paired testes, genital ducts, accessory glands, and penis. The accessory sex glands include the two seminal vesicles, the single prostate and the paired bulbourethral (Cowper's) glands. The testis is one of the most important organs of the male reproductive system. The two primary functions of the testis are production of sperm and synthesis of androgens. The emphasis of this histological practical will be on the microscopic structure of the testis with special reference to its parenchymal seminiferous tubules together with the interstitial cells (Leydig cells).

【Objectives】

1. To identify and describe:

A. the structure of the seminiferous tubules.

B. germ cells at different stages of spermatogenesis: spermatogenic cells (spermatogonia, primary spermatocytes, secondary spermatocytes, spermatids, spermatozoa); supporting cells (Sertoli cells); interstitial cells (Leydig cells).

2. To understand the main features of the tunica albuginea, interstitial tissue, tubuli recti and rete testis.

3. To understand the main features and functions of the epididymis, vas deferens (ductus deferens), prostate gland and seminal vesicle.

【Observation of tissue section】

1. Testis, H & E

An image of the testis at low magnification (Figure 17-1): Tunica albuginea is a thick layer of dense connective tissue in which are scattered a number of smooth muscle cells. Seminiferous tubules in cross and oblique sectional profiles, form the principal structure of the testis. Testicular interstitial tissue, composed of loose connective tissue is located between the seminiferous tubules.

An image of the testis under the high power lens (Figure 17-2): An enlarged view of seminiferous tubule (asterisk, Figure 17-2). Arrows indicate a distinct colony of interstitial (Leydig) cells in the testicular interstitial tissue. Leydig cells are either rounded or polygonal in shape with a centrally located nucleus and an eosinophilic cytoplasm rich in small lipid droplets (white arrow, Figure 17-2 and black arrow, Figure 17-3).

A high magnification image of a part of the wall of a seminiferous tubule shows various stages of spermatogenesis, and Sertoli cells (Figure 17-3). The latter are readily identified by the presence of a clear jagged or triangular shaped nucleus with a large, centrally positioned nucleolus. The spermatogonia (A, Figure 17-3) which are round or ellipsoid are relatively small cells, about 12μm in diameter. They are situated adjacent to the basal lamina of the ep-

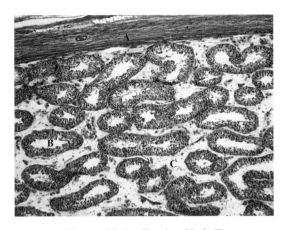

Figure 17-1　Testis, H & E

A: Tunica albuginea; B: Seminiferous tubule;

C: Interstitial tissue

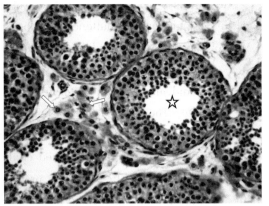

Figure 17-2　Testis, H & E

Asterisk: Seminiferous tubule; White arrows: Leydig cells

ithelium. The primary spermatocytes (B, Figure 17-3) are the largest cells within the seminiferous epithelium. They are spherical or ovoid in shape, about 16μm in diameter. The nucleus is usually characterized by the presence of chromatin (chromosomes) at various stages of the coiling process. Secondary spermatocytes are difficult to identify in sections of the testis because they are short-lived cells. The spermatids (C, Figure 17-3) may be distinguished by their small-sized (about 6μm) diameter and spherical in shape. Within the seminiferous tubules, the spermatids are close to the lumen. Spermatozoa (D, Figure 17-3) are long or tadpole-shaped cells in the lumen. Each spermatozoon is made up of a head, housing the nucleus, and a tail.

Tubuli recti are short straight tubules (white arrows, Figure 17-4). Each tubule segment connects the seminiferous tubules to the rete testis where the epithelium is abruptly transformed into simple cuboidal or columnar epithelium.

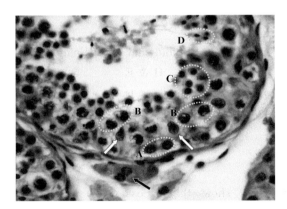

Figure 17-3　Seminiferous tubule, Testis, H & E

A: Spermatogonia; B: Primary spermatocytes;

C: Spermatids; D: Spermatozoa; White arrows:

Sertoli cells; Black arrow: Leydig cells

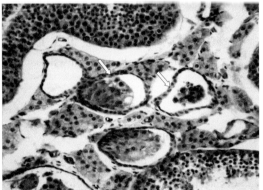

Figure 17-4　Tubuli recti, Testis, H & E

White arrows: Tubuli recti

Rete testis is a labyrinthine network of channels within the mediastinum. It is generally lined by a single layer of flattened or cuboidal cells, and is surrounded by connective tissue (Most of your slides do not show this two tubular segment).

2. Epididymis, H & E

The epididymis caps the posterior part of each testis. It is divided into three parts: head, body, and tail. The head consists of tightly coiled efferent ductules. The efferent ductules are lined by ciliated columnar epithelium. Note that most of your slides do not show this. The body and tail of epididymis are termed epididymal duct. Image of the epididymis under the low power lens (Figure 17-5) shows profiles of epididymal ducts in cross and oblique sections. Spermatozoa are aggregated in the lumen.

A high magnification image of the epididymal duct (Figure 17-6): The wall of the epididymal duct consists of a tall pseudostratified columnar epithelium surrounded by connective tissue and smooth muscle. The two major cell types of the epithelium rest on a basement membrane. The tall columnar cells show elongated, euchromatic nuclei, and long, apical stereocilia. The small, round basal cells resting on the basement membrane do not reach the luminal surface.

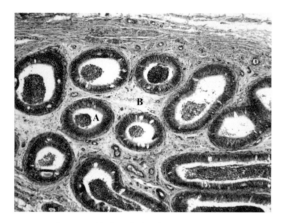

Figure 17-5   Epididymis, H & E

A: Epididymal duct; B: Connective tissue

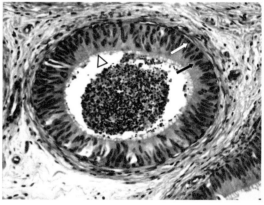

Figure 17-6   Epididymal duct, Epididymis, H & E

Arrowhead: Stereocilia (branched microvilli);
White arrow: Basal cell; Black arrow: Columnar cell

【Demonstration slides】

1. Vas deferens (Ductus deferens), H & E

A section of the ductus deferens (Figure 17-7) shows the mucosa which is lined by pseudostratified columnar epithelium with stereocilia (identified as branched microvilli under the electron microscope) and a lamina propria. The thick outer wall shows smooth muscle and collagen fibers.

2. Prostate gland, Masson trichrome stain

A high magnification image shows the prostate gland in section (Figure 17-8). Pseudostratified columnar epithelium, consisting of columnar cells and small basal cells, lines the secretory alveolus. Prostatic concretions (corpora amylacea) are in the alveolar lumen. A prominent fibromuscular stroma is in the adjacent areas.

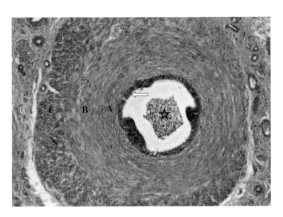

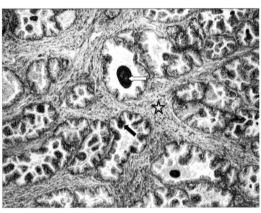

Figure 17-7   Vas deferens (Ductus deferens), H & E

White arrow: Epithelium; Asterisk: Spermatozoa; A: Inner longitudinal smooth muscle; B: Middle circular smooth muscle; C: Outer longitudinal smooth muscle

Figure 17-8   Prostate gland, Masson trichrome stain

White arrow: Prostatic concretion; Black arrow: Epithelium; Asterisk: Stroma

3. Seminal vesicle, H & E

A low power image of the seminal vesicle in section (Figure 17-9). The seminal vesicle is a small tortuous tubular organ. The mucosa is characterized by extensive folding, which is covered by a simple columnar epithelium. It rests on a thick layer of smooth muscle.

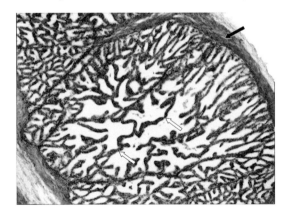

Figure 17-9   Seminal vesicle, H & E

White arrow: Mucosa folding; Black arrow: Smooth muscle

【**Questions and clinical points for discussion and integration**】

1. What is the difference in lymphatic drainage between the testis and scrotum?

2. Where is the site of vasectomy normally done?

3. Review the innervation of the male reproductive system.

4. What is blood-testis barrier? What is its functional significance?

5. How does Viagra work? What is the molecular mechanism of its action?

6. What are the clinical signs of prostatic hypertrophy?

7. Which cell organelle is well developed in the interstitial cells of Leydig?

8. Which biomarker is clinically used for prostatic screening, e. g. cancer, inflammation or hypertrophy?

9. What is the difference between "spermatogenesis" and "spermiogenesis"?

(周德山)

Chapter 18   Female Reproductive System

The female reproductive system consists of the internal reproductive organs (the paired ovaries and oviducts [uterine tubes], uterus and the vagina) and the external genitalia. Its functions are to produce female gametes (oocytes) and to hold a fertilized oocyte during its complete development until birth. The system also produces sex hormones. The ovaries and the uterus are the most important organs of the female reproductive system. Mammary glands are not classified as genital organs, but are functionally associated with them. The following are learning objectives for this histological practical class.

【Objectives】

1. To identify and describe:

A. the general organization of the ovary and the structure of the follicles; the primordial, primary and antral (secondary) follicles.

B. the structure of the uterus and histological changes of the endometrium through the menstrual cycle.

2. To understand and describe the main histological structure of the oviduct (uterine tube) and vagina.

3. To understand and describe the main histological structure of the mammary glands.

【Observation of tissue sections】

1. Ovary, H & E

Under the low power lens, the ovary is surrounded by the germinal epithelium and lying deep to this is the tunica albuginea. It is indistinctly divided into the cortex and the medulla. The ovarian cortex is composed of the connective tissue stroma that houses the ovarian follicles at various stages of development. The medulla consists of loose connective tissue with blood and lymphatic vessels as well as nerves.

Figure 18-1 is an enlarged view of the ovarian cortex under the high power lens. The germinal epithelium, covering the ovary, is a single layer of cuboidal cells. Immediately beneath this epithelium is the tunica albuginea, a layer of dense connective tissue. Groups of primordial follicles, each composed of a primary oocyte and surrounded by a single-layered of flattened follicular cells are distributed in the ovarian connective tissue (stroma). The primary follicle is composed of a primary oocyte surrounded by a unilayered or multilayered of cuboidal or columnar shaped-follicular cells. Between the primary oocyte and the follicular cells is the densely stained eosinophilic membrane, the zona pellucida.

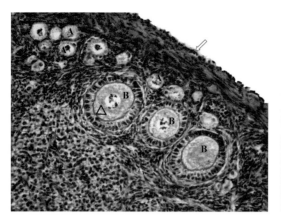

Figure 18-1   Ovary, H & E
White arrow: Germinal epithelium; A: Primordial follicles; B: Primary follicles; Arrowhead: Zona pellucida

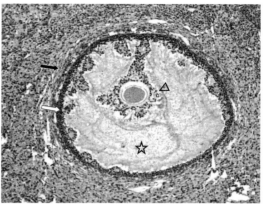

Figure 18-2   Secondary follicle, Ovary, H & E
Asterisk: Follicular antrum; Arrowhead:Cumulus oophorus; White arrow: Granulosa cells; Black arrow: Theca externa

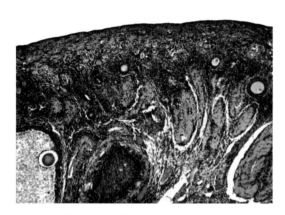

Figure 18-3   Ovary, H & E
A: Atretic follicles; B: Corpus albicans

This photo-image shows a secondary follicle (Figure 18-2). Once the multilaminar primary follicle displays the presence of one or more liquid containing follicular cavities of different sizes, it is known as the secondary or antral follicle. Cavities that appear in the granulosa layer will eventually coalescence to form one large cavity, the antrum (asterisk, Figure 18-2). The primary oocyte is surrounded by the zona pellucida, granulosa cells of the corona radiata and supported by cells of the cumulus oophorus (arrowhead). The remaining granulosa cells (white arrow, Figure 18-2) form the wall of the follicle and surround the large antrum. A theca externa (black arrow, Figure 18-2), composed of connective tissue surrounds the whole follicle.

Photomicrograph of the atretic follicles (A, Figure 18-3) characterized by the death of granulosa cells, many of them are seen loosely organized in the antrum; loss of the cells of the corona radiata; and the free floating oocyte within the antrum. The corpus albicans (B, Figure 18-3) shows scars of connective tissue that has replaced the corpus luteum after its involution.

2. Uterus (proliferative phase), H & E

A low power image shows the endometrium of the uterus (Figure 18-4). The wall of the uterine body and fundus is made up of an endometrium, myometrium, and adventitia or serosa (parametrium). The endometrium is lined by a simple columnar epithelium resting on a layer of supporting lamina propria. The myometrium, a thick muscular wall of the uterus, is composed of three layers of smooth muscle.

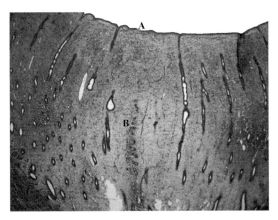

**Figure 18-4　Uterus（proliferative phase），
H & E**

A：Epithelium；B：Lamina propria；C：Myometrium

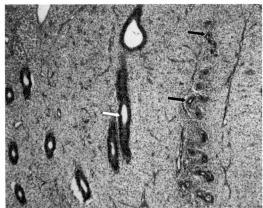

**Figure 18-5　Uterus（proliferative phase），
H & E**

White arrow：Uterine gland；Black arrows：Spiral arteries

　　Photomicrograph showing the endometrium at the early proliferative phase（Figure 18-5）. The uterine glands and spiral arteries are embedded in a lamina propria made up of loose connective tissue. The endometrium is relatively thin, and glands are simple and straight. The following image（Figure 18-6）is a low power photomicrograph showing the endometrium at the late proliferative phase. An enlarged image shows the endometrium at the late proliferative phase（Figure 18-7）. The thick endometrium shows a marked growth in glands and stroma. The concertina-like uterine glands are extremely tortuous or convoluted.

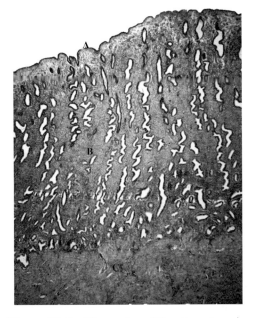

**Figure 18-6　Uterus（proliferative phase），
H & E**

A：Epithelium；B：Lamina propria；C：Myometrium

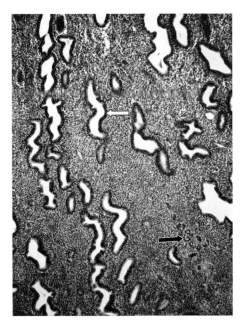

**Figure 18-7　Uterus（proliferative phase），
H & E**

White arrow：Uterine gland；Black arrow：Spiral arteries

3. Uterus (menstrual phase), H & E

A low photomicrograph shows the endometrium of the uterus at the menstrual phase (Figure 18-8). An enlarged image shows the endometrium during the menstrual phase that is characterized by the desquamation of the functional layer (Figure 18-9).

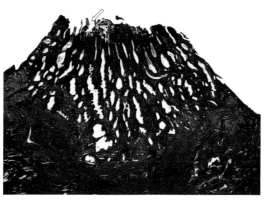

Figure 18-8   Uterus (menstrual phase), H & E

A: Endometrium; B: Myometrium; White arrow: Desquamation of the functional layer

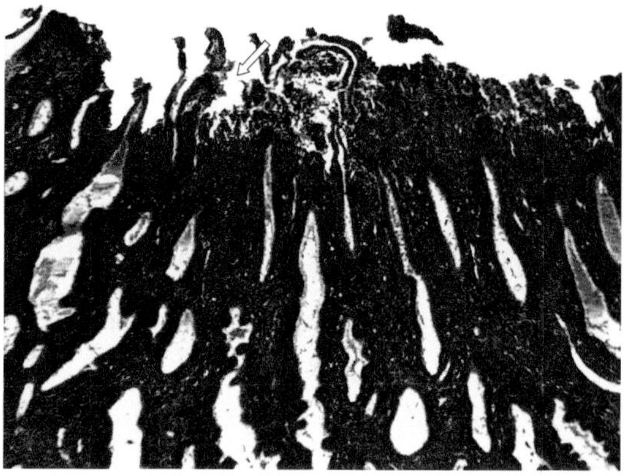

Figure 18-9   Uterus (menstrual phase), H & E

White arrow: Desquamation of the functional layer

【Demonstration slides】

1. Mature (Graafian) follicle, H & E

An image shows a mature (Graafian) follicle (Figure 18-10). On one side of the follicle is seen the oocyte which is surrounded by a thin layer of granulosa cells, the corona radiata. The oocyte and corona radiata protrude into the large follicular antrum. The antrum is delineated by a stratified epithelium of granulosa cells, which are enveloped by the theca interna and externa (Most of your slides do not show the mature follicle).

2. Corpus luteum, H & E

Light micrograph of a corpus luteum (Figure 18-11). After ovulation, the granulosa cells and the cells of the theca interna of the ovulated follicle reorganize to form a temporary endocrine gland called the corpus luteum, which is embedded within the cortical region. Many blood vessels (BV) filled with red blood cells are seen at the periphery.

3. Oviduct(Uterine tube, fallopian tube), H & E

Light micrograph of an oviduct in cross-section (Figure 18-12). The wall of the oviduct is composed of three layers: mucosa, muscularis, and serosa. The mucosa is characterized by many longitudinal folds. Question: What is its lining epithelium? The muscularis is composed of an outer longitudinal and an inner circular muscle layers.

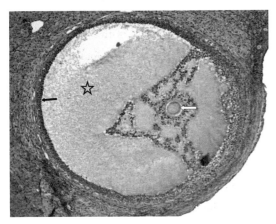

Figure 18-10　Mature (Graafian) follicle, Ovary, H & E

Asterisk: Follicular antrum; White arrow: Oocyte; Black arrow: Granulosa cells

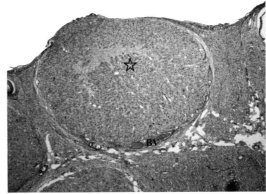

Figure 18-11　Corpus luteum, Ovary, H & E

Asterisk: Corpus luteum; BV: Blood vessels

4. Endometrium (secretory or luteal phase), H & E

Light micrograph of the endometrium at the secretory phase of the cycle at low magnification (Figure 18-13). Uterine glands are highly tortuous and have a serrated outline in section. The spiral arteries appear more coiled.

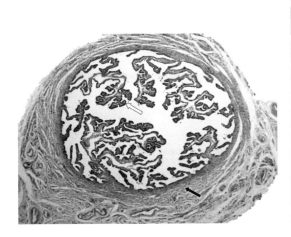

Figure 18-12　Oviduct, H & E

White arrow: Fold; Black arrow: Muscularis

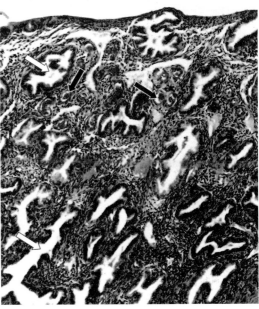

Figure 18-13　Secretory phase of the endometrium, H & E

White arrows: Uterine glands; Black arrows: Spiral arteries

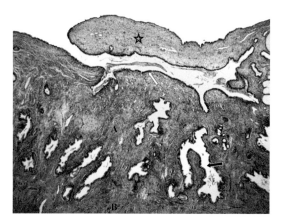

Figure 18-14　Uterine cervix, H & E

A: Mucosa; B: Smooth muscle; White arrow: Epithelium;
Black arrow: Cervical gland; Asterisk: Fold

5. Uterine cervix, H & E

Photomicrograph of the cervix (Figure 18-14). It differs in histological structure from the rest of the uterus. The lining of the cervical canal consists of a mucus-secreting simple columnar epithelium. The cervix shows few smooth muscle fibers and consists mainly of dense connective tissue in its walls. The mucosa of the cervix contains the mucous cervical glands, which are extensively branched.

6. Vagina, H & E

The wall of the vagina is composed of four layers: mucosa, submucosa, muscularis, and adventitia. The mucosa consists of epithelium and underlying lamina propria. The epithelium is characterized by nonkeratinized stratified squamous epithelium that lacks glands. Deeper in the lamina propria is submucosa rich in elastic fibers and thin-walled blood vessels (white arrows, Figure 18-15). A high power image of the vagina mucosa shows the cytoplasm of epithelial cells is clear or appears empty-looking because it was occupied by glycogen in the living but had been dissolved during histology slide preparation (Figure 18-16).

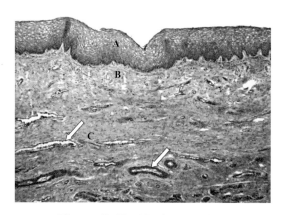

Figure 18-15　Vagina, H & E

A: Epithelium; B: Lamina propria; C: Submucosa;
White arrows: Blood vessels

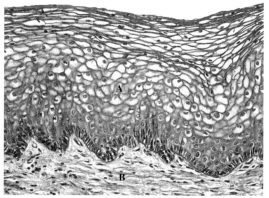

Figure 18-16　Vagina, H & E

A: Epithelium; B: Lamina propria

7. Resting (inactive) mammary glands, H & E

A low power photomicrograph of the mammary gland at resting state (Figure 18-17). The mammary gland is made up of 15 ~ 20 lobes separated by dense connective tissue and a substantial amount of adipose tissue. The parenchyma of each lobe is composed of numerous lobules; each lobule is composed of small ducts lined by a simple cuboidal epithelium.

8. Lactating (active) mammary gland, H & E

A low power light micrograph of the active (lactating stage) mammary gland (Figure 18-18). Identify the closely packed sac-like alveoli that synthesize and secrete milk. The lumen of the lactiferous duct is filled with a flocculent eosinophilic precipitate (milk components). Question: What is the mode of secretion by the alveolar cells?

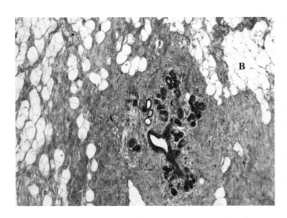

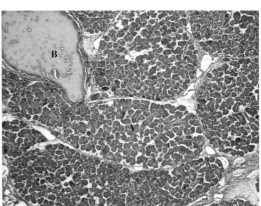

Figure 18-17　Resting mammary glands, H & E

A: Dense connective tissue; B: Adipose tissue; C: Lobule

Figure 18-18　Lactating mammary glands, H & E

A:Lobule; B: Interlobular duct

【Questions and clinical points for discussion and integration】

1. Describe the histological features of the fundus of the uterus.

2. Give an account of the histology of the ovary. What is the arterial supply to the organ?

3. Describe the cyclical histological changes of the endometrium through the menstrual cycle.

4. Where is the common site of cervical cancer? What procedure is being routinely used clinically for screening of cervical cancer?

5. The epithelial lining cells of the vagina are rich in glycogen. What is the functional significance of this?

6. How do you differentiate the vagina from the esophagus in histology sections?

7. What is ectopic fertilization?

8. Which hormone acts on the uterine wall smooth muscle?

9. What is the source of the hormone in the uterus?

10. What are the various stages of development of ovarian follicles? Describe the formation of a corpus luteum. What hormones are secreted by it?

(李娟娟)

Table of Slides